building bone vitality

A Revolutionary Diet Plan to Prevent Bone Loss and Reverse Osteoporosis

Amy Joy Lanou, Ph.D.

Michael Castleman

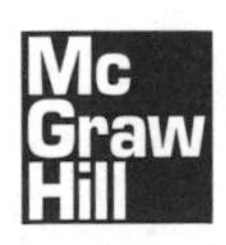

New York Chicago San Francisco Lisbon London Madrid Mexico City
Milan New Delhi San Juan Seoul Singapore Sydney Toronto

The McGraw-Hill Companies

Library of Congress Cataloging-in-Publication Data

Lanou, Amy Joy.
Building bone vitality : a revolutionary diet plan to prevent bone loss and reverse osteoporosis / Amy Joy Lanou and Michael Castleman.
p. cm.
ISBN 0-07-160019-1 (alk. paper)
1. Osteoporosis—Alternative treatment—Popular works. 2. Osteoporosis—Nutritional aspects—Popular works. I. Castleman, Michael. II. Title.

RC931.O73L42 2009
616.7′16—dc22 2008039786

To the four matriarchs in my family: my grandmothers, Dorothe Smith and Florence Stewart, the latter of whom suffered osteoporosis, and to my mothers, one by birth and one by marriage, Sandra L. Kinzie and Barbara Lee Smith, who instilled a love of vegetables and fruit and who model healthy bone maintenance lifestyles for their children and friends.

—Amy Joy Lanou

To the three most important women in my life: my mother, Mim Castleman, my wife, Anne Simons, and my daughter, Maya Castleman.

—Michael Castleman

2 3 4 5 6 7 8 9 10 11 12 13 14 15 16 17 18 19 20 21 22 23 24 DOC/DOC 0 9

ISBN 978-0-07-160019-4
MHID 0-07-160019-1

This book is printed on acid-free paper.

Contents

Foreword

THIS BOOK WILL CHANGE the way you think about bone density and osteoporosis. The weakening of bones is often viewed as a calcium deficiency, when actually it's an imbalance between calcium intake and excretion.

As nutrition professor Amy Joy Lanou, Ph.D., and noted medical journalist Michael Castleman eloquently reveal, diets rich in animal protein, including meat and dairy, add acid to the blood. This acid accelerates osteoporosis by depleting bones of calcium, phosphorus, and sodium.

As the authors recommend, the most effective way to prevent bone loss is a combination of daily walking and what they call *low-acid eating*—that is, predominantly fruits, vegetables, legumes, and soy products—with little, if any, meat, dairy, and fish and a modest amount of breads, cereals, and pastas.

For more than thirty years I have directed a series of clinical studies in collaboration with my colleagues at the nonprofit Preventive Medicine Research Institute and the University of California, San Francisco, showing that a similar regimen (when combined with stress management techniques such as yoga and meditation and psychosocial support) can often stop or even reverse the progression of coronary heart disease, diabetes, high blood pressure (hypertension), high cholesterol (hypercholesterolemia), prostate cancer (and, by extension, breast cancer), and other chronic diseases.

Many people believe that advances in medicine have to be high-tech and expensive. In our studies, we have used the latest high-tech medical technology to prove how powerful a plant-based diet, moderate daily exercise, and other simple, low-tech, low-cost interventions can be.

It's no coincidence that the program I recommend to prevent or even reverse coronary heart disease and other chronic diseases also helps prevent osteoporosis. It's the same program the National Cancer Institute recommends to prevent the most common types of cancer and that many other health authorities endorse for optimal health and well-being. The body is an elegant biological system. What's good for one part of it—for example, the heart and blood vessels—is also good for other parts, such as strengthening bone and helping to protect against fractures.

Lanou and Castleman have analyzed more than twelve hundred studies showing that (1) the United States and other countries that consume the most milk, dairy, and calcium have the world's *highest* fractures rates; (2) milk, dairy foods, and calcium supplements do not reduce fracture risk and in some studies *increase* it; and (3) a diet high in fruits and vegetables consistently improves bone mineral density and reduces fractures.

If you follow their advice, you're likely to reduce your risk of osteoporosis and fractures as well as enhancing your overall health and well-being. I wholeheartedly recommend *Building Bone Vitality*.

—Dean Ornish, M.D.

Founder and President, Preventive Medicine Research Institute

Clinical Professor of Medicine, University of California, San Francisco

Author, *Dr. Dean Ornish's Program for Reversing Heart Disease* and *The Spectrum*

Acknowledgments

THE AUTHORS GRATEFULLY ACKNOWLEDGE and thank:

- Their agent, Amy Rennert, and everyone at the Amy Rennert Literary Agency, Tiburon, California
- Their editors, Emily Carleton, Nancy Hall, Johanna Bowman, and Deborah Brody, and everyone at McGraw-Hill
- Their families and friends, who graciously put up with their bone obsession during the writing of this book
- And Neal Barnard, M.D.; T. Colin Campbell, Ph.D.; Simon Chaitowitz; Sophie Mills, Ph.D.; Dean Ornish, M.D.; Barbara Ramsey, M.D.; Keith Ray, Ed.D.; Anne Simons, M.D.; Louanne Cole Weston, Ph.D.; and Tania Winzenberg, Ph.D.

Introduction

An Evidence-Based Approach to Bone Health and Osteoporosis Prevention

We've been told all our lives to drink milk for strong bones. Many of us may even feel guilty when we don't consume our recommended three servings of dairy each day. In fact, we've been led to believe that we have a "calcium crisis" in the United States because many of us don't drink the requisite three glasses. The proposed solution? Drink more milk. Eat more yogurt and cheese. And to be sure we're getting enough calcium to protect our bones, take a calcium supplement.

But why do we think that milk, dairy foods, and calcium supplements prevent the broken bones (fractures) that osteoporosis causes? Because we've been told by our teachers, our doctors, and advertisers that we need lots of calcium to keep our bones strong as we age. And because every major U.S. health agency endorses daily consumption of milk and dairy: the surgeon general, the Centers for Disease Control and Prevention (CDC), the National Institutes of Health, and the Osteoporosis Foundation.

How do *they* know that the conventional dietary wisdom prevents osteoporosis and fractures? Perhaps because research has shown that osteoporotic bone contains less calcium than healthy bone. And because dairy has lots of calcium per serving. So the logical conclusion is to drink milk to get more calcium into the body. But what if all that dairy and supplemental calcium doesn't make it into bone or stay there?

Have you ever wondered why so many of us end up with brittle bones, height loss, and hip fractures as we age? Isn't it surprising that we have increased our overall dairy and calcium intake as a nation at the same time that our osteoporosis rates are skyrocketing? If milk and supplemental calcium are the answer, shouldn't hip fracture rates be *declining*?

It turns out that the conventional dietary wisdom on osteoporosis is just plain wrong. We'll show you that the great weight of the scientific evidence demonstrates that milk, dairy, and calcium pills neither strengthen bone nor reduce risk of fractures.

We present a new explanation of osteoporosis that has been hiding in plain sight in the medical literature for forty years. Since 1968, hundreds of studies have called the conventional dietary wisdom on osteoporosis into serious question. The clear majority of the best studies support an alternative explanation—low-acid eating.

We offer several safe, simple, effective, and low-cost diet and lifestyle suggestions that, unlike the conventional wisdom, actually strengthen bone and reduce fracture risk. Low-acid eating also helps prevent many other public health problems, among them, heart disease, cancer, stroke, and Alzheimer's disease.

We need to eat some calcium—but much less than recommended by U.S. health authorities. The best sources may surprise you—greens and beans. Low-acid eating paired with daily walking keep calcium in bones. That's the key: choose a dietary pattern and lifestyle that allows bone to absorb—and retain—dietary calcium.

You'll find that low-acid eating is quite simple. Eat two servings of fruit and/or vegetables at every meal and snack on fruit and vegetables. And cut down on—or eliminate—animal foods, and go easy on cereals, breads, and pastas. Pair this with walking (or other weight-bearing exercise) for at least a half hour a day from childhood to old age, and your risk of osteoporotic fractures plummets by 50 percent, a decrease most osteoporosis drugs can't match.

That's the solution to osteoporosis—and a safe, effective, low-cost prescription for health, vitality, and longevity.

Don't Take Our Word for It

We cite more than 1,200 studies. Synopses of studies discussed in Chapters 3 through 5 are listed in the appendixes. References to studies cited in the rest of the book can be viewed by visiting: BuildingBoneVitality.com. Abstracts of all studies we cite can be obtained for free from the National Library of Medicine (pubmed.gov). For downloading directions, see page 235. Or if you prefer, we'll send you the complete set of abstracts—1,536 pages of material. For details, see page 236.

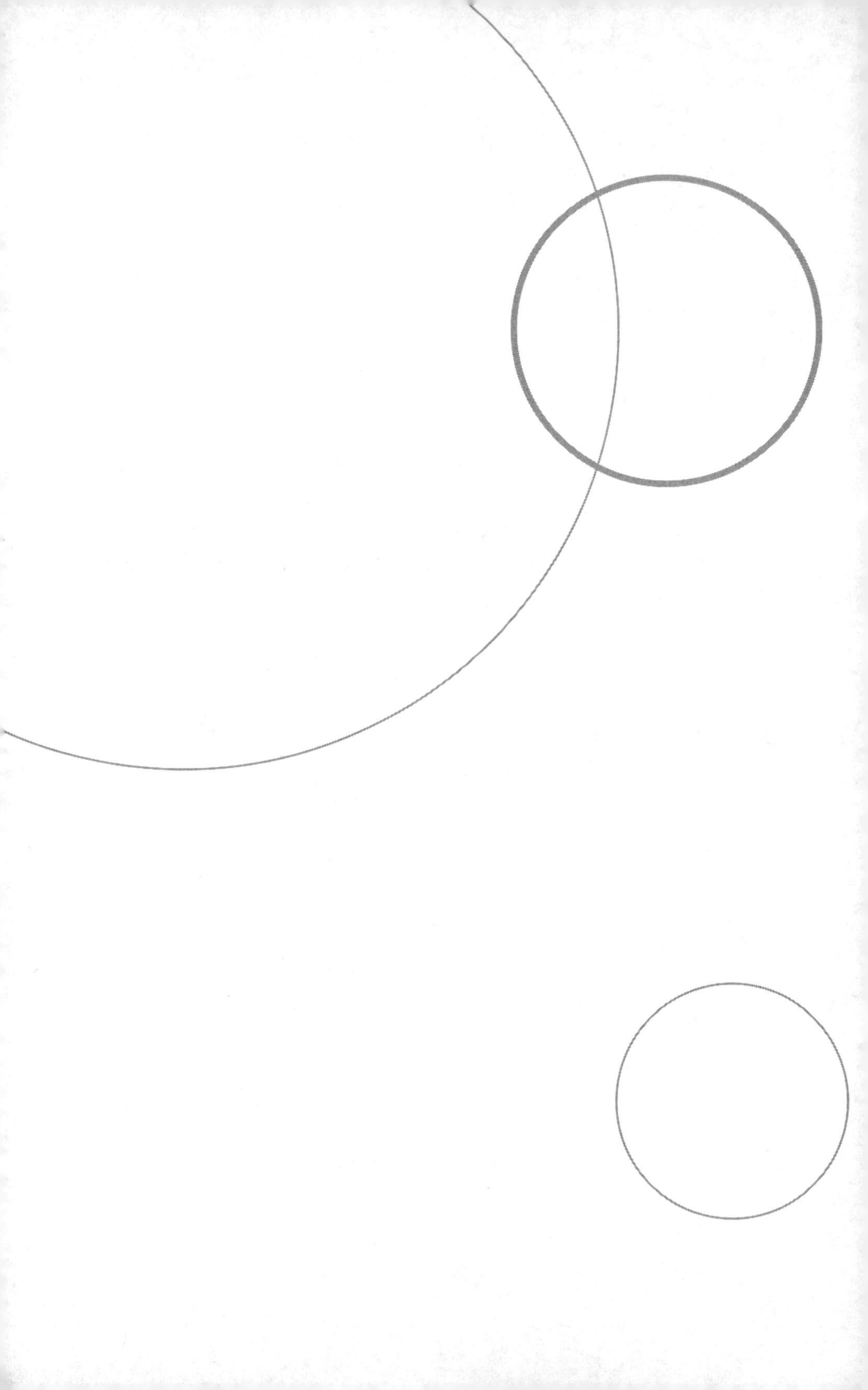

PART 1

Why the Calcium Theory Is Wrong

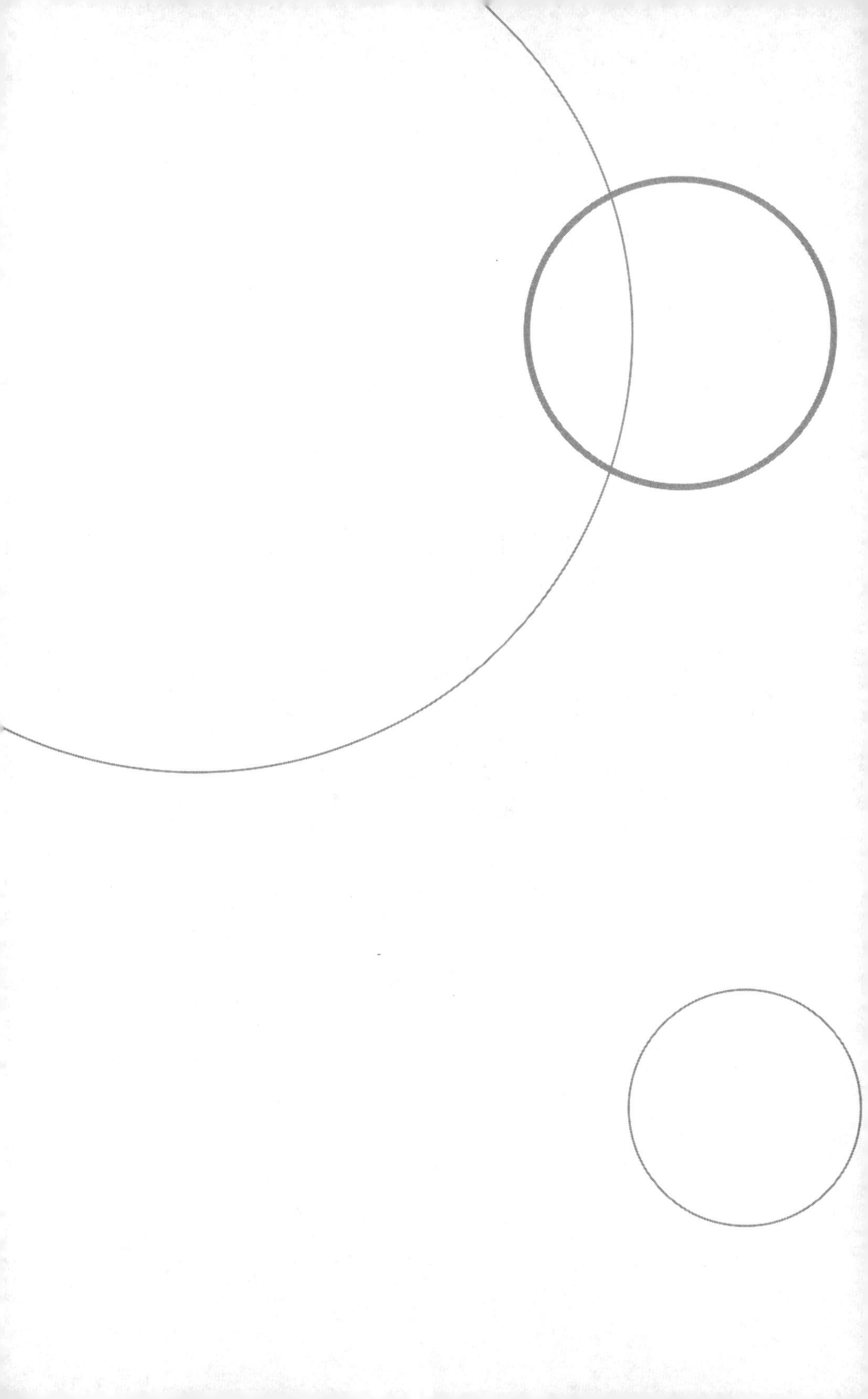

Countries That Consume the Most Milk, Dairy Foods, and Calcium Supplements Suffer the Most Fractures

Osteoporosis causes 1.5 million fractures a year in the United States, making it the nation's leading cause of broken bones. It causes millions more fractures worldwide. These fractures are painful, debilitating, costly, and, in the case of hip fractures, often life-threatening (see the sidebar "The Staggering Toll of Osteoporosis in the United States," on page 15). As a result, the U.S. government has declared 2002–2011 the National Bone and Joint Disease Decade.

News coverage often implies that twenty-first-century Americans suffer so many osteoporotic fractures because we enjoy much longer life spans than our ancestors. If you live long enough, that is, the disease is inevitable.

It isn't.

Rates of osteoporotic fractures vary tremendously around the world. Some countries have hip fracture rates many times greater than others. (These are "age-adjusted" rates, meaning that they compare people of the same age.) Since 1975, the year the medical literature became easily searchable by computer, four studies—published in 1985, 1992, 2000, and 2006—have documented osteoporotic hip fracture rates around the world. (See Tables 1.1–1.4.)

TABLE 1.1 1985, Mayo Clinic Researchers

Age-adjusted hip fracture rates per 100,000 population in women age 35 or older

Hip Fracture Rate	Location
421	Norway, Oslo
320	USA, Rochester, Minnesota
313	Indians living in Singapore
257	South Africa, Johannesburg (white)
237	Sweden, Malmo
232	USA, District of Columbia (white)
220	New Zealand (white)
213	Finland
202	Israel, Jerusalem (American- or European-born)
187	Netherlands
168	Israel, Jerusalem (native-born)
142	Israel, Jerusalem (Asian- or African-born)
142	United Kingdom, Oxford
119	USA, District of Columbia (African-American)
105	Croatia (low-calcium region)
104	New Zealand (Maori)
87	Hong Kong
59	Singapore (Chinese)
44	Croatia (high-calcium region)
24	Singapore (Malay)
14	South Africa, Johannesburg (black)

SOURCE: Melton, J. L. "Epidemiology of Fractures," in *Osteoporosis: Etiology, Diagnosis, and Management*, B.L. Riggs and L. J. Melton (eds.), Raven Press: New York, 1988.

TABLE 1.2 1992, Yale Researchers

Age-adjusted rates per 100,000 population for women over age 50

Hip Fracture Rate	Country	Data Collected During
221	Norway	1978–79
214	Sweden	1981
192	Sweden	1965–80
190	Norway	1983–84
188	Sweden	1972–78
165	Denmark	1971–76
165	Denmark	1973–79
149	Norway	1972–73
145	United States (white)	1974–79
131	United Kingdom	1983
122	Sweden	1950–60
119	New Zealand	1973–75
118	United States (white)	1980
118	United Kingdom	1977
116	United Kingdom	1978–79
111	Finland	1980
97	Finland	1970
93	Israel	1957–66
91	United Kingdom	1975
88	Netherlands	1967–79
77	United Kingdom	1954–58
76	Ireland	1968–73
72	Finland	1968
60	United States (nonwhite)	1980
52	Former Yugoslavia	1968–73
46	Hong Kong	1965–67
42	Spain	1974–82
34	United States (nonwhite)	1974–79

continued

TABLE 1.2 1992, Yale Researchers (continued)

Hip Fracture Rate	Country	Data Collected During
28	Former Yugoslavia	1969–72
22	Singapore	1955–62
21	Former Yugoslavia	1968–73
7	South Africa (black)	1957–63
3	Papua New Guinea	1978–82

SOURCE: Abelow, B. J. et al. "Cross-Cultural Association Between Dietary Animal Protein and Hip Fracture: A Hypothesis," *Calcefied Tissue International* (1992) 50:14.

TABLE 1.3 2000, University of California, San Francisco, Researchers

Age-adjusted rates per 100,000 population for women over age 50

Hip Fracture Rate	Country
199	Germany
187	Norway
172	Sweden
165	Denmark
148	Argentina
139	New Zealand
130	Switzerland
125	Australia
120	United States
120	Portugal
117	United Kingdom
113	Crete
110	Canada
94	Finland
77	France
76	Ireland
76	Israel

TABLE 1.3 2000, University of California, San Francisco, Researchers (continued)

Hip Fracture Rate	Country
69	Hong Kong
67	Japan
65	Spain
61	Netherlands
57	Italy
57	Chile
47	Saudi Arabia
34	Former Yugoslavia
27	Malaysia
22	Singapore
12	South Korea
8	South Africa
5	Thailand
3	New Guinea
3	China
1	Nigeria

SOURCE: Frassetto, L. A. et al. "Worldwide Incidence of Hip Fracture in Elderly Women: Relation to Consumption of Animal and Vegetable Foods," *Journal of Gerontology: Medical Sciences* (2000) 55:M585.

TABLE 1.4 2006, Tehran University Medical School, Iran, Researchers

Age-adjusted rates per 100,000 population for women over age 50

Hip Fracture Rate	Country	Data Collected
764	Norway	1998
710	Sweden	1991
554	United States	1989
504	Australia	1996
497	Taiwan	2000

continued

TABLE 1.4 2006, Tehran University Medical School, Iran, Researchers (continued)

Hip Fracture Rate	Country	Data Collected
484	Hong Kong	1998
470	Greece	1992
432	Singapore	1998
418	England	1998
402	Kuwait (non-Kuwaitis)	1995
399	Germany (former West)	1996
355	Germany (former East)	1996
346	Switzerland	1992
316	Kuwait (Kuwaitis)	1995
297	Japan	1994
262	Thailand	1998
213	Malaysia	1998
168	Brazil	2000
165	Iran	2003
86	China, Beijing	1996
80	Morocco	2002

SOURCE: Moayyeri, A. et al. "Epidemiology of Hip Fractures in Iran: Results from Iranian Multicenter Study on Accidental Injuries," *Osteoporosis International* (2006) 17: 1252.

These studies take different approaches and use different source studies to calculate fracture rates. As a result, the four studies' findings differ. Nonetheless, their results are strikingly similar. By and large, the highest rates of hip fracture cluster among Western countries: North America, Europe (especially northern Europe), Australia, and New Zealand. Hip fracture is much less of a problem in Africa, Asia, and South America.

Clearly, osteoporosis is not inevitable. What, then, accounts for the vast differences worldwide?

Got Milk?

In common parlance, a theory is a hypothesis, an educated guess. In science, however, a theory is a widely accepted explanation for a great deal of observed reality, such as the theory of evolution or the germ theory of illness. The conventional wisdom on diet and osteoporosis might be called the calcium theory of bone health.

Our health authorities insist that the calcium triumvirate—drinking milk, eating dairy foods, and taking calcium pills—is the best dietary approach to preventing osteoporosis. But if the calcium theory were correct, we would expect countries that consume the most milk, dairy, and calcium to have the world's *lowest* hip fracture rates.

They don't. They suffer the world's *highest* rates of hip fracture.

According to the Food and Agriculture Organization of the United Nations, Americans and Western Europeans consume much more milk and dairy than Asians and Africans. Think of all the milk, cheese, yogurt, frozen pizza, and ice cream in the typical American refrigerator. Think of all the cheeseburgers, milk shakes, and lattes Americans consume. Think of Swiss cheese, French Brie and Camembert, Irish cheddar, Dutch Gouda, and Danish blue, not to mention all the cheese in Italian food. Finally, North Americans and Europeans take the lion's share of the world's calcium supplements. Yet hip fracture rates are highest in the United States and Western Europe.

Meanwhile, most people in Asia consume little or no milk after weaning. Many Asian cuisines—Chinese, Japanese, Thai, and Vietnamese—contain *no* milk or dairy products. The calcium theory predicts that elderly hips in these countries should be snapping like dry twigs. Yet their rates are among the world's lowest.

Put another way, total calcium consumption among women in China, Peru, Sri Lanka, and many other non-Western countries is only about 500 milligrams a day, yet fracture rates are very low. Meanwhile, calcium consumption in the United States and Western Europe is close to 1,000 milligrams a day, but in these countries older women face an epidemic of osteoporotic fractures.

The only Asian country with a high fracture rate is Indians living in Singapore (the 1985 study). Indian food is the only Asian cuisine that contains cheese.

In the four worldwide studies, the only glimmer of hope for the calcium theory is the 1985 study's findings about fracture rates in two regions of Croatia. One consumes much more calcium than the other. As the calcium theory predicts, the high-calcium region has a substantially lower rate of hip fracture. But a closer look at this study reveals that the Croatian trial investigated not just hip fractures but also osteoporotic wrist fractures, and the two regions' rates of wrist fracture are *the same*. If the calcium theory were correct, we would expect the high-calcium region to have low rates of both types of fractures. There are other reasons to question this study as well, discussed in Chapter 3.

There's no getting around it: the countries that consume the most calcium have the highest rates of osteoporotic fractures. The United Nations World Health Organization calls this the *calcium paradox*. Osteoporosis authorities have been scratching their heads about it for more than twenty years. They have suggested several possible explanations.

Vitamin D Deficiency

Vitamin D boosts the body's ability to absorb calcium. That's why most milk in the United States is fortified with vitamin D.

Vitamin D is unique among nutrients. It's the only vitamin we make ourselves. Although it's possible to obtain small amounts of vitamin D from food (fish liver oils and tuna, cod, halibut, sea bass, sable, and swordfish), most is produced by the skin when exposed to sunlight. Vitamin D deficiency was not an issue when our ancestors were hunter-gatherers. They spent most of their days outdoors. Nor was it a problem during the period from around 6000 B.C. until late in the nineteenth century, when the vast majority of people farmed. They, too, spent much of their lives outdoors.

But over the past 150 years, as urbanization has moved increasing numbers of people indoors for much of the day, vitamin D deficiency has become a problem, particularly for older people, the age group that spends the least time outdoors. In addition, fear of skin cancer has led to widespread use of sunscreens, which reduce the skin's ability to synthesize vitamin D. As a result, many people are deficient in this vitamin and don't absorb as much calcium as they might.

The Scandinavian countries lie far north of the equator. They get very little daytime sunlight for much of the year. Perhaps, experts speculate, vitamin D deficiency explains their high rate of fractures and the calcium paradox.

But it doesn't.

If vitamin D deficiency explained the high fracture rates in Scandinavia, we would expect the bone strength of Scandinavian-type people, white people, to increase as we move south from the Baltic. We would expect fracture rates among whites to decrease. They don't. Consider the 1985 study. Israel lies much closer to the equator than Scandinavia. Yet American- or European-born Israelis suffer hip fractures at rates almost as high as those in Sweden and Finland.

Consider Washington, DC. It receives much more daytime sunlight than Scandinavia, but according to the 1985 study, white people in the nation's capital suffer as many hip fractures as Scandinavians. In the 1992 report as well, whites in the United States have hip fracture rates similar to Scandinavia.

Or consider the 2000 study: Germany and the Netherlands are located at more or less the same latitude, but Holland's hip fracture rate is less than one-third of Germany's.

Finally, consider the 2006 study: the former East and West Germany lie at the same latitude, but hip fractures are more of a problem in the West than the East.

Perhaps vitamin D deficiency has something to do with worldwide differences in hip fracture risk. But by itself, vitamin D deficiency provides no compelling explanation for these differences or for the calcium paradox.

Exercise

Weight-bearing exercise plays a key role in bone strength and fracture resistance. Meanwhile, Americans are notoriously sedentary. According to the Centers for Disease Control and Prevention (CDC), only 48 percent of Americans get the recommended thirty to sixty minutes of regular, moderate exercise (walking, biking, swimming, gardening, and so forth) every day. Some osteoporosis experts blame a sedentary lifestyle for America's high rate of hip fracture. This makes sense—until we look at the rates worldwide.

Consider Saudi Arabia. In Saudi society, women are largely confined to their homes. Many are not allowed to appear on the street without a male relative escort, and by U.S. standards their educational, employment, and activity opportunities are quite limited. It's hard to see how the typical Saudi woman could get much exercise. Yet, in the 2000 study, Saudi women's risk of hip fracture is less than half that of American women.

Now consider Singapore, a technologically advanced, densely urbanized country filled with motor vehicles where most people live in high-rise apartment towers and do as little physical labor as most Americans. In all four studies, Singaporeans' risk of hip fracture is considerably lower than Americans'.

Perhaps differing rates of exercise have something to do with worldwide differences in hip fracture risk. But by itself exercise provides no compelling explanation for these differences or for the calcium paradox.

Race/Genetics

Many studies show that hip fracture rates vary substantially among the races, with whites having higher rates than Africans or Asians. As a result, some researchers have suggested that racial genetic differences govern bone strength.

At first glance this appears plausible. Consider the 1985 study. Whites and African-Americans living in Washington, DC, have similar sun exposure, but the whites have almost twice the risk of hip fracture. The situation is similar for whites and the native Maori in New Zealand and for European- versus African-born Israelis. In every case the whites suffer considerably more hip fractures.

But if race determines bone strength, we would expect all whites, all Asians, and all Africans to have approximately the same fracture risk. This is not the case. In all four studies, Asian residents of Hong

Kong have higher rates than other Asians—in the 2000 study more than twenty times the rate in China. In addition, African-American women in Washington, DC, have much greater hip fracture risk than black African women.

Finally, in the 2000 study, Nigerians have a tiny hip fracture rate, just 1 per 100,000, much less than any figure for African-Americans. Meanwhile, the ancestors of most African-Americans were taken from the area around Nigeria. This happened only four hundred years ago, nowhere near long enough for genetic differences to have developed. In other words, Nigerians and African-Americans come from similar genetic stock, but African-Americans suffer much more osteoporosis.

While race may play some role in fracture risk, by itself it offers no compelling explanation for worldwide differences or for the calcium paradox.

Epidemiology: A Science of Insights—and Limits

As the four studies show, osteoporosis is *not* an epidemic in much of Asia, Africa, or Latin America. But it has reached epidemic proportions in the United States and much of Europe. As a result, it has attracted interest from epidemiologists, who focus on the big picture—the forest, not the trees.

Epidemiology's strength is its ability to discover associations. One of its greatest triumphs was the discovery of the association between smoking and lung cancer. An association may show scientific researchers where to look for cause-and-effect relationships, but it never *proves* a cause-and-effect link on its own. Epidemiologists first noticed an association between smoking and lung cancer during World War II. But it took hundreds of studies over twenty years before the U.S. surgeon general finally declared unequivocally in 1964 that smoking causes lung cancer.

Sometimes associations that look causal turn out not to be. Men living near the Gulf Coast have unusually high cancer rates. Does living near the Gulf of Mexico cause cancer? No. The men with cancer work in the many petrochemical plants in that area. It's long-term exposure to petrochemicals, not simply residing near the gulf, that explains those cancer rates.

While associations are always intriguing, they must be approached skeptically. Before even mentioning cause and effect, we must ask whether the association is *real.*

The association between high rates of fractures and milk, dairy, and calcium certainly look real. After all:

- We're not dealing with just one study, but four.
- The four studies were conducted by four different groups of investigators on two continents.
- They consider fracture rates in dozens of countries.
- They were conducted not at just one point in time but over a period of twenty-one years.
- Finally, despite their differences, all four studies share the same basic finding: the countries that consume the most milk, dairy, and calcium suffer the most hip fractures.

The association appears real.

In fact, based on the four studies, one might even speculate that milk, dairy foods, and calcium supplements *cause*—or at least contribute to—fractures. But this would be jumping to a conclusion. It's possible that, like the association between a Gulf Coast address and cancer, some other factor might explain *both* high calcium intake and our epidemic of osteoporotic fractures.

To determine what causes osteoporosis, what prevents it, and the role that milk, dairy foods, and calcium play in the condition, we have to go beyond the big picture. Epidemiology isn't enough. We need to focus more narrowly on the people who suffer osteoporotic fractures and how they differ from those who don't. Researchers use four types of studies to do this. We discuss them—briefly—in the next chapter.

The Staggering Toll of Osteoporosis in the United States

- Currently 10 million Americans over age fifty have osteoporosis —8 million women and 2 million men. Another 34 million have osteopenia, bone mineral density considerably below normal but not low enough to be diagnosed as osteoporosis.
- Every year 1.5 million Americans, overwhelmingly women, suffer an osteoporotic fracture.
- Every year osteoporosis causes 300,000 hip fractures; 700,000 vertebral fractures; 250,000 wrist fractures; and 300,000 other fractures.
- Currently, 40 percent of white women over age fifty suffer a hip, wrist, or vertebral fracture at some point.
- Currently, one woman in six—17 percent—fractures a hip during her lifetime. That risk is as high as women's risk of breast, uterine, and ovarian cancer *combined*. Six percent of older men suffer hip fractures—more than develop prostate cancer.
- Osteoporotic fractures result annually in 800,000 emergency room visits, 500,000 hospitalizations, and 2.6 million doctor visits.
- By themselves, osteoporotic fractures are rarely fatal. But they often trigger a downward spiral of deteriorating health that soon results in death. Compared with people with intact hips, during the three months after an osteoporotic hip fracture, risk of death *quadruples*.
- During the year after a hip fracture, 25 percent of people die.
- Only one-third of people who break a hip because of osteoporosis ever regain their independence. Those who survive hip fractures often become disabled. Almost half require canes or walkers.
- A broken hip is a leading cause of placement in nursing homes. Within a year of hip fracture, 20 percent of people—one in

continued

five—must move to a nursing home. Osteoporosis accounts for 180,000 nursing home placements per year.

- In 2002, in the United States alone, medical care for osteoporotic fractures cost $18 billion. That figure is so large that it's difficult to imagine.
- As the 77 million Americans of the baby boom generation grow older, the osteoporosis epidemic is predicted to grow. By 2020, experts predict that osteoporosis will increase 40 percent to 14 million Americans and that half of Americans over fifty will have weak bones at serious risk for fractures. By 2040, the number of hip fractures could double to 600,000 per year.

Not Just a Woman's Disease

Many people believe that osteoporosis is a woman's disease, that it's possible but rare in men. Not so. Plenty of men develop osteoporosis and suffer fractures.

- Italian researchers estimate that men suffer 25 percent of all osteoporotic hip fractures.
- Australian researchers analyzed every fracture in one small city over a five-year period in people over age sixty. Approximately one-third of the fractures occurred in men.
- After osteoporotic hip fractures, men's death rate is higher than women's.

Women suffer more osteoporosis than men for several reasons:

- **Longevity.** Women live longer than men. Osteoporotic fractures are most prevalent among the oldest people. Compared with men, many more women live past eighty. Even if men and women over eighty suffer fractures at the same rate, the population of women is much larger, so many more fractures occur in women.

- **Genetics.** In all racial and ethnic groups, men have greater bone mineral density (BMD) than women.
- **Hormones.** The female sex hormone estrogen suppresses bone loss. After menopause, estrogen declines and bone loss increases. That's why osteoporotic fractures become common after menopause. Compared with women who experience normal menopause, those who enter menopause early (usually because of ovary removal or chemotherapy) experience earlier bone loss and fractures at younger ages. (More on estrogen in Chapter 16.)
- **Exercise.** Men tend to be more physically active than women. Exercise builds and strengthens bone. (More on this in Chapter 13.)

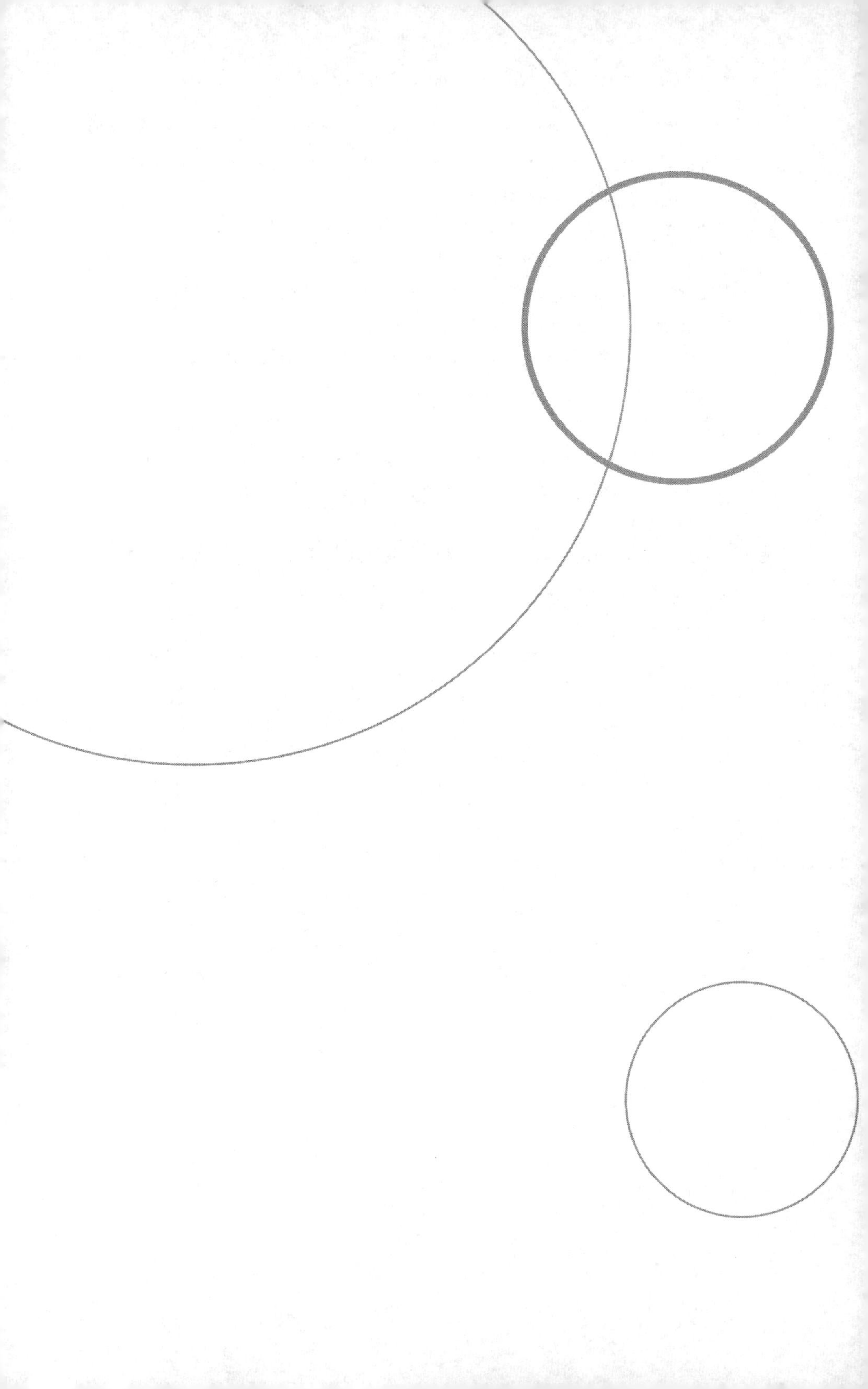

Why Some Osteoporosis Studies Should Be Taken More Seriously than Others

THE NATIONAL INSTITUTES of Health spend about $100 million a year on osteoporosis research. That's a fortune. But in a nation of 300 million, it's just 33 cents per person annually—next to nothing. Such research funding limits are not unusual. Scientists in every field struggle with chronically inadequate funding. As a result, researchers must squeeze the maximum bang out of every buck.

But what if money were no object? What would the best possible study to discover the risk factors for osteoporotic fractures look like?

- It would use people, not animals. No experimental animals—rats, dogs, monkeys—consume milk after weaning. And no animals eat the variety of foods humans eat. So the best study of human osteoporosis would use human subjects, a *clinical trial.*

- It would include every baby born in the world over many years or at least a huge subset of all births.
- It would track their diets, lifestyles, and everything else about them as they grew from infancy through adulthood into old age.
- It would also ask some participants to change their lives in certain ways and make sure they did.
- Then it would record every fracture that everyone suffered and use a vast array of supercomputers to correlate those fractures with the subjects' diets, lifestyles, and thousands of other aspects of their lives.

Of course, it would be far too costly and time-consuming to follow hundreds of thousands or tens of millions of people for their entire lives. Not even the most intrusive police state could keep such close tabs on everyone. And neither the agencies that fund research nor the scientists who conduct it want to wait seventy-plus years to release results.

Prospective Trials: Moving Forward in Time

Fortunately, to investigate osteoporosis and other health issues scientists don't need to study billions of people over a lifetime. They can approximate what happens to all of us by using smaller—but carefully chosen—population samples.

Perhaps you've heard of the Framingham Heart Study. In 1948, researchers recruited five thousand residents of Framingham, Massachusetts, into what quickly became a landmark study of heart disease, ongoing for more than sixty years. In addition to heart disease, Framingham data have been used to study osteoporosis risk. Or maybe you've heard of the Nurses' Health Study. Launched in the 1970s, it continues to track the diet, lifestyles, and health of ninety thousand women nurses—including their risk of osteoporotic fractures.

When the Framingham and Nurses' studies were launched, the researchers examined the participants and surveyed their diets, lifestyles, medications, and other aspects of their lives. Since then they have regularly reexamined and resurveyed the participants.

Researchers survey participants periodically over time so they can see how people live as the years pass. Such studies are called *prospective trials. Prospective* means "moving into the future." The researchers started with a large group and have followed them over time.

There are several types of prospective studies. The Framingham and Nurses' trials are *cohort studies.* Researchers start with a large group that has something in common, a cohort, and keep tabs on them. *Population studies* follow even larger groups. *Experimental studies* typically use smaller groups.

In addition, prospective trials can be organized in several ways. *Observational studies* track the group over time. *Interventional trials* ask some of the group to change some aspect of their lives—for example, by taking a calcium supplement. They become the intervention group. The rest do not make the change, or they take a dummy treatment (placebo). They become the control group. If a study has a control group, it's called a *controlled trial.* Then the researchers track what happens to both groups over time and look for differences in outcome, such as fracture risk.

Observational trials have produced many important results, but it's impossible to determine what causes what simply by tracking a large group over time. Interventional trials are better. They allow researchers to see if the intervention causes any effect. Some Framingham and Nurses' Health Study trials have been observational. Others have been interventional, typically involving subsets of the total group.

The gold standard of clinical trials is the *randomized, double-blind, controlled trial (RDBCT)*. These studies have intervention and control groups. To eliminate possible researcher bias, the participants are assigned to their group at random. In addition, the trial is blinded. When the participants don't know which group they're in, but the researchers do, the study is known as *single-blind.* When neither the participants nor the researchers know who's in which group, it's called *double-blind.*

To investigate things like the effects of new drugs, randomized, double-blind, controlled trials are best. But they're impractical for studying common health problems like fracture risk, heart disease, or cancer because these conditions don't strike that many people over the typical study's duration. Only .5 percent of the American population (one in two hundred) has an osteoporotic fracture each year—a number big enough to warrant close study but too small for RDBCTs.

It's very expensive and time-consuming to launch RDBCT trials. It's more cost-effective to study fracture risk using population or cohort studies. Indeed, both the Framingham and Nurses' studies—and many other cohorts around the world—have supplied information on fracture risk. Some have been observational. Others have used subsets of cohorts or populations for interventional studies. (For the sake of brevity throughout this book we don't distinguish among the various types of prospective trials. We just call them "prospective.")

But because prospective trials are closest in design to real life, they are also considered to produce the best, most credible scientific evidence. Unfortunately, not many prospective trials get funded. Although they're much less costly than RDBCTs, it costs a fortune to track tens of thousands of people for many years, especially in interventional trials. Our search of the medical literature identified sixty-three prospective trials published since 1975 dealing with dietary risk factors for osteoporotic fractures.

- **Advantages of prospective trials:** Closest to real life. Most credible results.

- **Disadvantages:** Expensive. Take many years. Large numbers of participants must be followed.

Retrospective and Cross-Sectional Trials: Looking Back in Time

An alternative approach is to look back in time through what are called *retrospective*, or *case-control*, studies. In retrospective trials, the researchers begin with people who have already suffered osteoporotic fractures; these are the cases. Then they recruit demographically similar people who have not; these are the controls. They survey both groups' diet and lifestyle, analyze how they differ, and see if any differences can explain the two groups' differing fracture rates.

Retrospective studies produce results much faster than prospective trials. They start with people who have suffered fractures, so the researchers need not wait years for fractures to occur. In addition, retrospective studies can yield statistically significant findings using fewer subjects, sometimes as few as a couple dozen.

But retrospective trials are still very expensive. The researchers must find the cases and balance them with carefully matched controls—demographically similar people. Our search of the medical literature since 1975 turned up fifty-eight retrospective trials of dietary risk factors for osteoporotic fractures.

Unfortunately, retrospective trials have a major—and unavoidable—flaw. Compared with prospective studies, they're less likely to reflect what happens in real life because they rely on participants' *memories* of events that may have happened many years earlier. In a prospective trial, researchers might ask, "How many glasses of milk have you consumed in the last week?" You might be off by a little, but how much less accurate do you think your response would be if a researcher asked, "How many glasses of milk have you consumed during the past year [or five, ten, or even fifty years]?"

Study results are only as valid as the data used to compile them. Retrospective trials' dependence on participants' long-term memories makes them less credible than prospective trials. In addition, memory plays tricks, especially when surveys ask about diet and health. People generally underestimate consumption of items considered harmful, notably cigarettes and alcohol. They also tend to overestimate intake of items presumed to be good for health, such as—you guessed it—milk. People who participate in osteoporosis studies might overestimate their milk intake, especially their consumption as children, the time when everyone assumes milk matters most. Statisticians have mathematical ways to minimize the impact of recall errors, but they can't eliminate the errors altogether.

Finally, in retrospective trials, the purportedly "matched" controls may not bear much resemblance to the cases. Controls may match in gender, age, general health, and geographic location. But if they don't match in occupation, income, religion, marital status, alcohol intake, and leisure activities, how similar are they? You have to match many variables to have truly similar groups. Of course, as the number of matched variables increases, so does the expense. As a result, some studies' "matched controls" are more matched than others'.

Finally, we have the *cross-sectional* trial. Think of these studies as snapshots. Cross-sectional trials look at the subject of interest—fractures, for example—at one point in time. Researchers conducting a cross-sectional trial might ask "How many people in our cohort have osteoporotic fractures right now?" The answer reflects the number of people who have suffered fractures in the *recent past*, so cross-sectional trials look somewhat back in time. (For convenience, throughout this book we consider cross-sectional trials retrospective.)

Over the years, retrospective trials have produced many important findings. But compared with prospective trials, scientists agree they are less credible.

- **Advantages of retrospective trials:** Quicker than prospective trials. Require fewer participants.

- **Disadvantages:** Still very expensive. Reliance on memory is an inherent problem. Less credible than prospective trials.

Bone Mineral Density Studies

Given the high cost of both prospective and retrospective trials, in the 1980s osteoporosis researchers set their sights on finding a quick, easy, objective measure of bone strength—one that didn't cost much, didn't depend on recall, and didn't require huge numbers of subjects or eons to come up with meaningful findings. They found it in bone mineral density (BMD), the amount of calcium and other minerals contained in bone. They reasoned:

- More than 99 percent of the body's calcium is found in teeth and bones.
- Bone is approximately 40 percent calcium. (The rest is other minerals and collagen, which is largely protein.)

- As osteoporosis develops, BMD declines.
- And very low BMD is a clear, strong risk factor for fractures.

Using this logic, it wasn't much of a leap to infer that if BMD increases, fracture risk should decrease. In 1993, the United Nations World Health Organization changed the definition of osteoporosis from having suffered a fracture to having a BMD below certain statistical benchmarks. Since then, tens of millions of women have had the x-ray that determines bone mineral density (dual-energy x-ray absorptiometry, or DXA or DEXA), and BMD has become synonymous with bone strength and fracture resistance.

In BMD studies, researchers test subjects' bone mineral density and then provide some intervention, such as a high-dairy diet or calcium supplements. After a while, BMDs are retested to see if the intervention had any effect.

BMD studies are by no means cheap. But they are easier, quicker, and much less expensive than either prospective or retrospective fracture trials. As a result, the vast majority of studies dealing with diet and osteoporotic fracture risk have focused on BMD. We found 406 BMD studies published since 1975, more than three times the combined total of prospective and retrospective diet-and-fracture trials.

Unfortunately, BMD research has two serious problems. Bone mineral density is a second rate test, a poor predictor of fractures. More on this in Chapter 9. And BMD research does not deal directly with the real downside of osteoporosis, fractures. It's one step removed from fractures. As a result, scientists consider BMD studies less credible than prospective and retrospective trials.

- **Advantages of BMD studies:** Cheaper, faster, and easier than prospective and retrospective trials.

- **Disadvantages:** Don't deal with fractures. More removed from real life than retrospective or prospective trials. Assume incorrectly that as BMD increases, so does fracture resistance.

Meta-Analyses

In medical research, the more participants, the better. As the number of participants increases, the findings become more believable. Consider two studies of fracture risk, one involving fifty subjects, the other fifty thousand. They produce different findings. Which would you believe? But with research funding always so scarce, many researchers can afford to study only small groups and wish they could afford larger ones.

Enter the statisticians. In the 1970s they came up with meta-analysis, a mathematical way to combine small clinical trials as though they'd all been part of one big one. A meta-analysis can make ten trials of a hundred people look like one trial of a thousand—with the larger number of participants increasing the results' credibility.

In addition, when small studies produce disparate results, meta-analysis can often reconcile them and produce a clearer conclusion.

But from the start, critics voiced objections:

- Meta-analyses aren't "real" studies. They don't focus on observed reality; only on other studies.
- They're only as good as the studies they amalgamate. If the studies in the meta-analyses are flawed, so is the meta-result.
- While statistics play an important role in all biomedical research, as statistical machinations become more elaborate, scientists become more skeptical.
- Finally, some meta-analyses of osteoporosis studies deal only with fracture research, while others combine fracture and BMD trials. Such amalgamations may muddy the waters.

Nonetheless, since 1975, more than fifteen thousand meta-analyses have been published dealing with an enormous number of medical issues, and initial doubts have been replaced by general (though still sometimes grudging) acceptance.

We found fifteen meta-analyses of dietary risk factors for osteoporotic fractures.

- **Advantages of meta-analyses:** Combining small studies increases the credibility of the findings. Where the results of small studies differ, meta-analysis can produce a single conclusion.

- **Disadvantages:** Meta-analyses don't deal directly with fractures. Reflect real life less than retrospective and prospective trials.

When "Significant" Isn't

To recap, since 1975 clinical trials of dietary risk factors for osteoporotic fractures include 63 prospective trials, 58 retrospective trials, 406 bone mineral density studies, and 15 meta-analyses.

Many of these studies show that milk, dairy foods, and calcium pills do, indeed, increase BMD and reduce fracture risk. But many others find that the conventional dietary wisdom makes no difference to either BMD or fractures. In fact, some show that as people consume more milk, dairy, and calcium pills, fracture risk *increases.* (More on this in the next chapter.)

Why do studies differ? If something is true, shouldn't all studies reach the same conclusion? They should. But they don't—for two reasons:

- Life is complex, messy, and unpredictable.
- Studies differ in design, quality, subjects, and scientific rigor.

That's why it's a big mistake to put much faith in any single study. The best insights come from examining *all* the research and considering the total weight of the evidence—including the studies' scientific credibility.

While the studies go both ways on milk, dairy, and calcium for fracture prevention, enough trials have supported the accepted wisdom so that the vast majority of news stories have repeatedly flashed the same headline: "New Study Shows Calcium Helps Bone."

Unfortunately, the news media rarely emphasize the type of study—prospective, retrospective, BMD, or meta-analysis. And they rarely discuss how the type of study relates to the believability or accuracy of its findings. In the news media, all research carries the same weight. If it makes the news, it must be important. And every time the headline reads "New Study Shows Calcium Helps Bone," the story inevitably explains that milk, dairy, and calcium strengthen bone *significantly.*

Interesting word, *significant.* In common parlance, it means "important." When meteorologists announce that a storm is significant, we prepare for its arrival. When the president makes a significant policy announcement, it's viewed as important. And when one person becomes another's significant other, we know they matter a great deal to each other.

But in science, *significant* means something entirely different. It means *statistically* significant. Statistical significance is complicated. But basically it means there's less than a 5 percent chance—less than one chance in twenty—that the study's results are a fluke. That's *all* it means. It doesn't mean the findings matter. They might, of course. But many research results are both statistically significant and trivial. Results can be statistically significant but not matter in the real world.

Which brings us back to the different types of osteoporosis studies. Of the four—prospective, retrospective, BMD, and meta-analysis—which are most likely to be *significant,* as in important in the real world where Americans suffer 1.5 million osteoporotic fractures a year? The fracture trials—prospective, retrospective, and the meta-analyses.

As noted earlier, the BMD studies are less important because they don't deal with fractures. If we want to develop insights into what really matters—fractures—we must focus on the fracture studies.

That's what we've done in Chapters 3, 4, and 5. We've delved into all 141 fracture studies published since 1975. We've already shown that the four worldwide surveys provide no support for the calcium theory. The same goes for the fracture trials. The weight of the evidence from the diet-and-fracture studies shows that *milk, dairy, and calcium supplements do not reduce the risk of osteoporotic fractures.*

That's right. Only 47 of the 141 studies (33 percent) show that milk, dairy, and calcium (even with added vitamin D) produce any significant—that is, *statistically significant*—drop in fracture risk. And when reductions occur, they are modest. Nineteen clinical trials (13 percent) are inconclusive. Meanwhile, 75 of the 141 trials (54 percent) show that the accepted wisdom is just plain wrong—that milk, dairy, and calcium do not reduce fracture risk.

Bottom line: Only one-third of clinical fracture trials support the calcium theory. Two-thirds do not. The evidence runs *two to one against the conventional wisdom.*

In politics, when a candidate wins 60 percent or more of the vote, pundits call it a landslide. By this yardstick, the calcium theory loses by a landslide, 33 to 67 percent. Once you've reached the end of Chapter 5, we think you'll agree that milk, dairy foods, and calcium supplements have little, if anything, to do with fracture prevention.

Medical News Reporting: The Tyranny of "The Latest Study"

The news media report what's new. Nothing wrong with that. But in addition to their blind spot about the credibility of the studies they cover, media devotion to what's new—the latest study—institutionalizes a lack of perspective that does not serve the public health.

One week the latest study shows that beer causes cancer, coffee causes heart disease, or whatever. The next week, the next study shows the opposite. Over time, instead of becoming informed, the public becomes chronically confused.

Media fixation on the latest study also gives the impression that it's the only one that matters, that the latest study somehow *cancels out* all previous research. It doesn't. The latest study is simply

continued

one of many. No single study is ever definitive. What counts is the weight of the evidence across *all trials*.

In fairness, news organizations occasionally produce in-depth reports that go beyond the latest study and look at the weight of the evidence. But this is the exception, not the rule.

In this book, we explore *all* the evidence—*every* published study our exhaustive search found on risk factors for osteoporotic fractures. It's possible that we missed a few. But we found more than a thousand.

The latest study is just one pixel on a big screen. It takes hundreds of pixels for the true picture to emerge. The only way to get to the bottom of osteoporosis is to explore the total weight of the evidence. That's what we have endeavored to do.

Milk, Dairy Foods, and Calcium Supplements by Themselves or in Any Combination Do Not Prevent Fractures

THE DIETARY MANTRA for the calcium theory is drink milk, eat yogurt and cheese, and take a daily calcium supplement. But the evidence shows that milk, dairy foods, and calcium (800 to 1200 mg/day) by themselves or in any combination do not prevent fractures. We found eighty-six studies published since 1975:

- Twenty-four (28 percent) support the calcium theory. They show that as consumption of milk, dairy foods, and calcium supplements increases, fracture risk falls.
- Forty-seven studies (54 percent) show that milk, dairy, and calcium pills do not prevent fractures. Curiously, two show that as milk and dairy intake rise, fracture risk *increases*.

By almost two to one—54 percent of trials to 28 percent—the conventional wisdom just doesn't hold water.

The remaining fifteen studies (17 percent) are inconclusive. They show that milk, dairy, and calcium reduce fracture risk at some skeletal sites but not others. Or they do so in some people but not others. Or that any risk reductions are not statistically significant—that they may well be chance findings. The inconclusive reports must be credited to the "no effect" side because they show no benefit for calcium. They might. But "maybe" isn't good enough. To be counted as having an effect, the treatment must show *clear benefits.*

Bottom line: two dozen studies (28 percent) support the accepted wisdom, and sixty-two (72 percent) do not. By more than two to one, the research resoundingly refutes the calcium theory. The contrast is even more startling when you look closely at the design, duration, and size of these studies:

- Only ten of the studies showing that milk, dairy, and calcium prevent fractures are prospective—the most credible design—compared to twenty-three (more than twice as many) of the trials that dispute the conventional wisdom.

- The prospective studies showing that milk, dairy, and calcium reduce fractures last up to fourteen years and average seven, compared to a much longer twenty-two years and average of eight for those refuting the calcium theory.

- The prospective studies showing that milk, dairy foods, and calcium supplements reduce fractures averaged 3,101 participants, compared to a four-times-greater average of 13,283 for those that refute the calcium theory. The largest trial supporting milk, dairy, and calcium involves 11,798 subjects. Seven of the trials refuting the conventional wisdom had more participants. Compared with the largest study supporting milk, dairy, and calcium, the largest no-benefit study is *seven times larger.* If milk, dairy, and calcium really reduce fracture risk, how is it possible that studies of 77,761;

72,337; 60,689; 43,063; and 39,787 people followed for an average of eight years don't show any benefit?

Not only do more than twice as many of the studies refute the calcium theory than support it, but more of those refuting studies were of the highly credible prospective design, they were longer-term, and they followed a lot more individuals. The weight of the evidence points to only one reasonable conclusion: milk, dairy foods, and calcium supplements do not reduce risk of osteoporotic fractures.

Wait! Isn't Simple Addition Just Too Simple?

Some critics may claim that it's scientifically unsound to simply tally up the studies for and against milk, dairy, and calcium. They might contend that we need an army of biostatisticians to delve deeply into the data and decide what the evidence shows.

The weight of research evidence can be determined in several ways. Adding up studies as we have is one valid approach—one that has been used by scientists for decades. Every study we cite has been conducted by university researchers. Every one has been published in a peer-reviewed scientific journal. And the total number we refer to is a large number—86 trials of milk, dairy, and calcium for fracture prevention in this chapter and more in Chapters 4 and 5, for a total of 140 studies.

Another valid approach is to conduct meta-analyses. In our tally, we've included the four that have investigated milk, dairy foods, and calcium supplements. Not one supports the conventional wisdom.

But it's true that simply adding up studies *doesn't* go far enough. An army of biostatisticians *should* tackle the dietary risk factors for osteoporosis, conducting the most rigorous super-meta-analysis ever attempted.

We believe, in fact, that the National Institutes of Health should fund such an analysis. Every year, osteoporosis costs the United States $18 *billion*. One of our colleagues, who does meta-analyses on bone-related topics as part of her research explained that a super-meta-analysis of the sort we propose here would likely cost less than $100,000. Even if a super-meta-analysis cost close to $200,000, that would represent less than a tiny fraction of 1 percent of just one year's cost of the disease. Isn't that worth it?

We're confident that such an investigation would confirm our refutation of milk, dairy foods, and calcium supplements. In the meantime, it's perfectly valid to tally up the studies that have been done so far. (See Appendix A for more information about the studies.)

More on the Croatia Study

Recall from Chapter 1 that in the 1985 study of worldwide hip fracture rates, the findings from Croatia appear to support the calcium theory. Residents of the region that consumed more milk and dairy had the lower rate of hip fractures. But the two regions' rates of wrist fractures were the same. That's why, in Appendix A, we list this study—Matkovic, 1979—as inconclusive.

In addition, this retrospective study ranks low on measures of scientific credibility:

- It involved only a hundred people from each region—very small numbers.
- Half of each region's participants were in their forties, and half were in their seventies. They were all asked to recall their lifetime milk and dairy consumption, a tall order. The researchers tried to minimize recall errors by interviewing participants twice, one year apart. But if you ask people who are seventy-four about their lifetime calcium consumption, and you ask the same people the same question when they're seventy-five, how much more believable are their answers?

We don't deny the results of the Croatian study. But a great deal more evidence—and much better evidence—shows that milk and dairy foods do not protect against osteoporotic fractures.

Calcium Intake During Childhood Does Not Prevent Fractures at Any Stage of Life

CLEARLY, MILK, DAIRY, and calcium don't reduce fracture risk in adulthood. However, the most rapid bone development occurs from birth to age twenty-five. Defenders of the conventional wisdom say that adulthood may be too late to load up on calcium—you have to do it during childhood and adolescence, when bones are still growing.

Children's skeletal development is a research focus for one of us (AJL). In 2005, in an article published in the journal *Pediatrics*, she and her coauthors reviewed all the research on calcium and dairy products as they relate to bone health in children. They found thirty-seven scientifically rigorous reports. Ten showed that milk, dairy, and calcium supplements increase bone mineral density in children. But twenty-seven—almost three times as many—showed no bone-health benefits from dietary calcium and supplements. In addition, in the ten studies giving calcium thumbs up, the benefits were so small that fracture prevention at any age appeared highly unlikely. The conclusion: "Neither increased consumption of dairy products nor total dietary calcium consumption has shown even a modestly consistent benefit for child or young adult bone health."

Australian researchers came to the same conclusion in a 2006 meta-analysis in *BMJ* (formerly the *British Medical Journal*) of nineteen studies of calcium supplementation in children: "The small effect of supplementation is unlikely to reduce the risk of fracture, either in childhood or later life to a degree of major public health importance."

These two papers include studies of both fractures and bone mineral density. In the rest of this section, we focus exclusively on the end point with the most public health impact, fractures.

We found thirteen studies published since 1975 that explore the effects of childhood milk, dairy, and calcium consumption on fractures throughout life. Four of the thirteen focus on the impact of childhood calcium consumption on later adult osteoporotic fractures.

- Two (50 percent) show that childhood calcium intake reduces adult fracture risk.
- Two (50 percent) show no later-life fracture-preventive benefit.

The rest of the studies—nine trials—focus on young people's calcium intake as it affects *non*osteoporotic fractures during childhood, adolescence, and young adulthood.

- Four of these studies (44 percent) show that consuming lots of milk, dairy foods, and calcium during youth reduces risk of fractures before adulthood.
- Five studies (56 percent) show that calcium during childhood makes no difference to childhood or young adult fractures.

This evidence makes no compelling case in favor of childhood calcium intake for prevention of fractures at any age. The score:

- Six studies (46 percent) show that childhood milk, dairy, and calcium intake reduce later fracture risk throughout life.
- Seven (54 percent) show no benefit.

Some might criticize our inclusion of the childhood fracture studies because they are nonosteoporotic. But a cornerstone of the conventional wisdom is that milk, dairy foods, and calcium during childhood are *absolutely essential* to building strong bones. If that's true, shouldn't calcium have some effect pretty quickly? It doesn't.

One of the trials in favor of milk and dairy asked Cincinnati-area women over age fifty how much they consumed starting when they were *just five years old*. Would you trust your own estimate of how much milk you drank at least forty-five years ago? A lousy study. But we did not discard it just because it contradicts our position. Even including this study, the final score is seven trials to six against the calcium theory.

Finally, one of the no-benefit studies, an Australian report involving 209 cases and 207 controls, shows that high intake of dairy products during youth is associated with an *increased risk* of hip fracture in later life.

Bottom line: there is no compelling evidence that childhood milk, dairy, and calcium consumption reduce fracture risk at any stage of life. (See Appendix B for more information about the studies.)

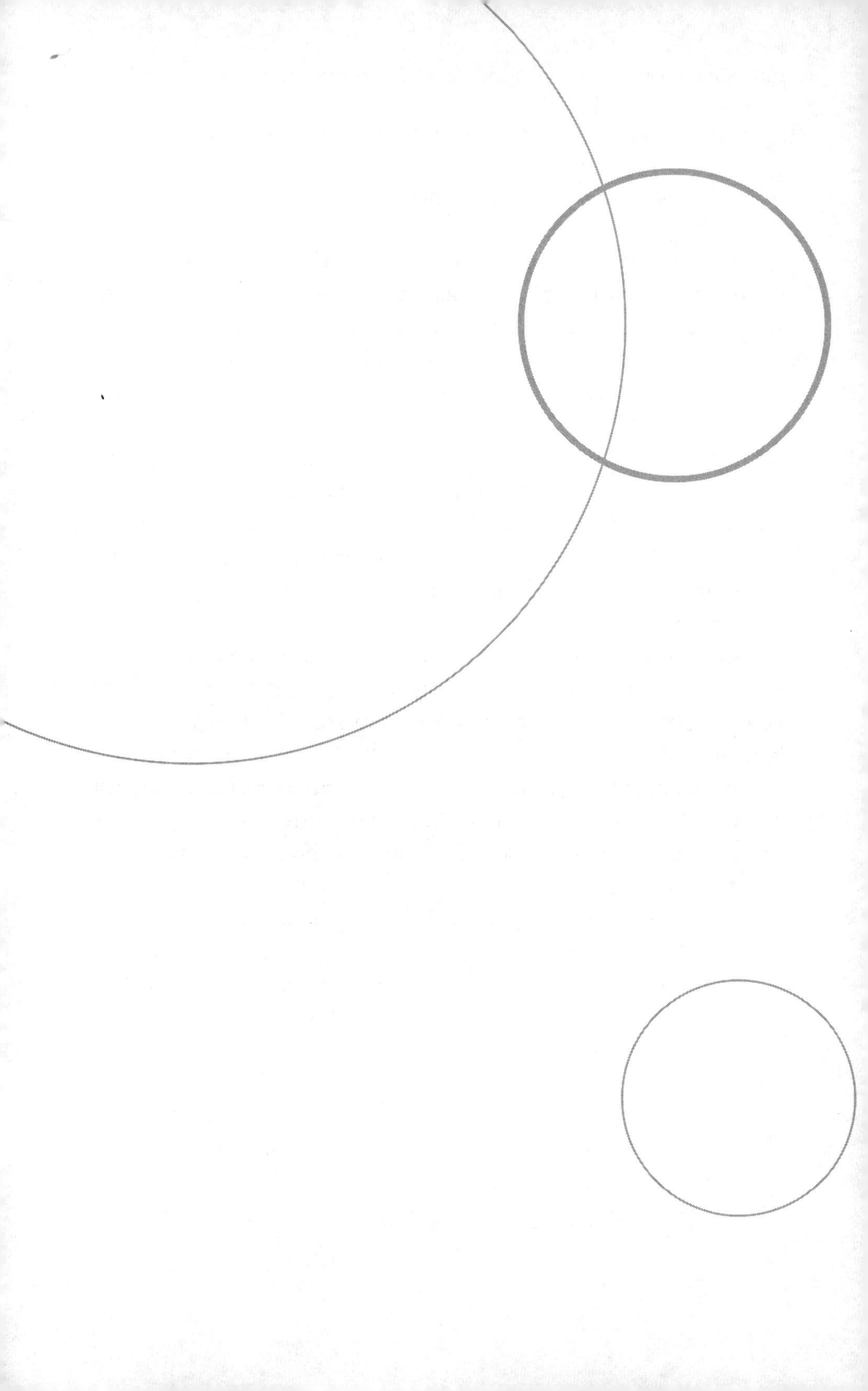

Vitamin D with or Without Calcium Prevents Few if Any Fractures

We are hardly the first to point out the weakness of the calcium theory. Over the past thirty years, the researchers who have conducted the dozens of studies showing that calcium provides no bone-building benefits have vocally challenged it, saying that it needed to be amended or abandoned. Defenders of the calcium theory countered that milk, dairy, and calcium are not enough. Many people are vitamin D deficient. Calcium must be combined with vitamin D so more of the mineral gets into bone.

We found thirty-seven studies published since 1975 that have investigated the effects of vitamin D with or without supplemental calcium on fracture risk. Doses ranged from 400 to 800 international units per day by mouth, or more by injection.

- Seventeen trials (46 percent) show statistically significant fracture prevention.
- Three (8 percent) are inconclusive.
- Seventeen studies (46 percent) show no benefit.

Again, the inconclusive reports must be credited to the "no effect" side because they show no benefit for vitamin D. By a score of twenty to seventeen, vitamin D fails. Once again, the accepted explanation doesn't hold up.

However, vitamin D represents the best showing for the (modified) conventional wisdom. Exclude the inconclusive trials and vitamin D ekes out a tie, seventeen to seventeen. Should we give the vitamin the benefit of the doubt? Three factors argue against this.

The Epidemiology

Recall that people living near the equator get much more vitamin D from sun exposure than people living in Scandinavia. If vitamin D reduces fracture risk, we would expect Scandinavian-type people, white people, who live south of Scandinavia to have lower fracture rates. They would get more sun and make more vitamin D. But recall from Chapter 1 that there is no consistent reduction in fracture risk among whites living near the equator. Vitamin D may play a role in osteoporosis prevention, but based on worldwide hip fracture epidemiology, it's clearly no cure.

The Prospective Trials

Of the seventeen studies that show benefit for vitamin D with or without calcium, ten are prospective. They involve 80 to 72,337 participants and average 8,976. They last from 1.5 to 18 years and average 4.2. In other words, the studies that support vitamin D involve large numbers of subjects and last long enough to produce credible results.

However, a larger number of prospective trials, thirteen, shows no benefit. These trials look just as credible. They involve 50 to 60,698 participants and average 12,949—more than the trials on the other side. They last from 1.2 to 11 years, averaging 3.8—a bit less than the pro–vitamin D research but still long enough to produce credible results, particularly since several of these reports focus on residents of nursing homes, people at very high risk of fracture. By a score of thirteen to ten, the best evidence tilts *against* vitamin D.

Now let's consider the largest, longest prospective trials. Only one study showing benefit for vitamin D involves more than 10,000 people. That study involves 72,337 postmenopausal women tracked for eighteen years. It shows that the vitamin by itself (no calcium) reduces fractures 37 percent. That looks pretty impressive—a huge number of women followed for a very long time, with fractures reduced by more than one-third.

But among the prospective trials showing no benefit, three involve more than 10,000 people. We have 36,282 postmenopausal women followed for seven years, 41,837 women tracked for three years, and 60,689 followed for eleven years. Again: big numbers followed for long periods. Yet *none* of these trials shows *any* reduction in fractures. If vitamin D is really effective, don't you think a study of 60,689 elderly women followed for eleven years would show *some* benefit? It doesn't.

The Effect Size

The results of the vitamin D studies are all over the map. Fracture reductions range from zero to 69 percent. In cases like this, meta-analyses are useful. By mathematically combining trials with very different results, statisticians can estimate the arguably real effect.

Nine meta-analyses have been published. Seven support vitamin D. Two show no benefit. Averaging them all together, it appears that vitamin D by itself or with calcium reduces fracture risk about 17 percent.

Seventeen percent. That's not much—especially in light of osteoporotic fracture rates around the world. Compared with the United States, many countries have rates *more than 70 percent lower.*

Few Asians or Africans take vitamin D or calcium supplements. Yet even without them, their fracture risk is substantially lower than that of Americans, Canadians, Western Europeans, Australians, and

New Zealanders who drink milk, eat dairy foods, and take calcium and vitamin D. Whatever the Asians and Africans are doing, it works substantially better than the best the calcium theory has to offer—even with added vitamin D.

Finally, the vitamin D research contains an important lesson. There's more to fracture prevention than just milk, dairy, and calcium.

When the Next Study Shows That Milk, Dairy, Calcium, or Vitamin D Prevents Fractures . . .

After this book is published, new diet-osteoporosis studies are sure to be published. No doubt, some will support the calcium theory. This should come as no surprise. Since 1975, forty-seven trials have supported milk, dairy, calcium, and vitamin D, more than one per year.

However, the next trial supporting milk, dairy, calcium, and vitamin D shifts the weight of the evidence only slightly. The next pro-calcium study makes the score forty-*eight* in favor and ninety-three against. The clear weight of the evidence will continue to refute the calcium theory.

With ninety-three studies showing the conventional wisdom worthless, it would take one more than that number—*ninety-four trials*—for milk, dairy, calcium, and vitamin D to account for the majority of trials. That would require *forty-nine* new studies supporting the conventional wisdom and none against.

For the conventional wisdom to claim the same two-to-one margin that now opposes it would require *192 new studies* in favor and none against.

In other words, the next study in support of milk, dairy, calcium, and vitamin D changes nothing. It would take an avalanche of research in support of the conventional wisdom—and no new studies opposed to it—to make a compelling case for milk, dairy, calcium, and vitamin D.

Several of the vitamin D studies show a significant drop in fracture risk when people take the vitamin all by itself—*without any calcium.*

It turns out that vitamin D is not the only noncalcium nutrient that helps build bone. There are many others. There's also an easy, safe, tasty, affordable way to consume all of them. More on this in Chapter 9. (See Appendix C for more on relevant studies.)

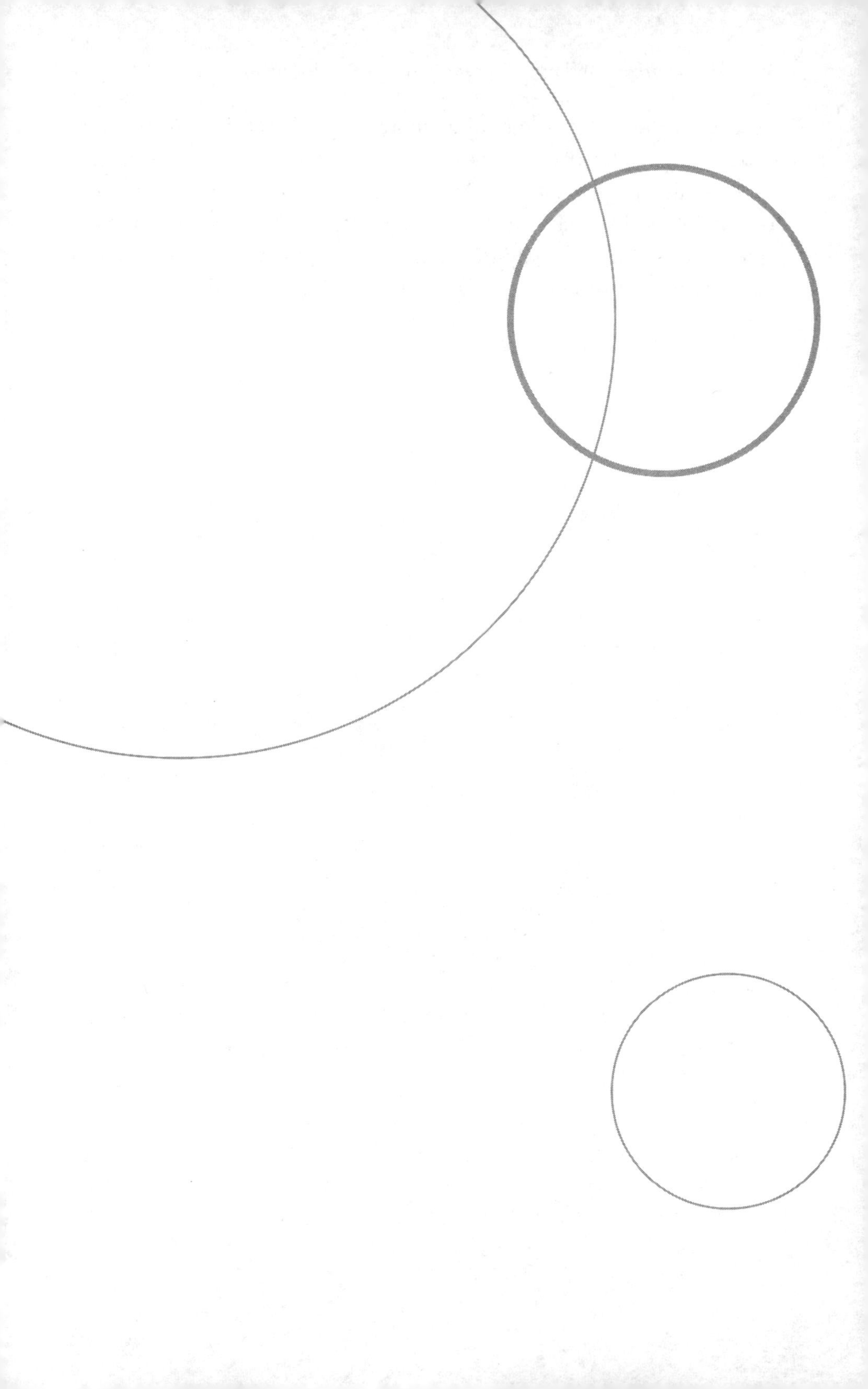

The Final Score: We Need a Theory That Works

IF A SPORTS team compiled a record of forty-seven wins, seventy-five losses, and eighteen ties, the players and fans would feel terrible. Forty-seven, seventy-five, and eighteen. That's what the calcium theory (even with vitamin D) has compiled over the past thirty-plus years.

Actually, the accepted explanation's record is even worse. How many trials truly support it? Just 47 of 140 trials (34 percent). Twice as many studies, 93 of 140 (66 percent), make no compelling case for the conventional wisdom. The trials line up *two to one against* milk, dairy, and calcium, even with vitamin D. If students answered just 34 percent of test questions correctly, they would fail miserably.

Meanwhile, compared with the rate of osteoporotic fractures in the United States, many other countries have rates more than 70 percent lower—using little, if any, milk, dairy foods, and calcium and vitamin D supplements.

The calcium theory—the conventional wisdom—is a failure. One hundred forty-one studies over more than three decades involving more than five hundred thousand participants and lasting for up to twenty-two years simply make no case for the notion that milk, dairy, and calcium, even with vitamin D, offer anything approaching a workable solution for osteoporosis.

Finally, it looks like milk and dairy might actually be *part of the problem.* The countries that consume the most milk and dairy have the world's highest fracture rates. And some large prospective trials show that as consumption of milk and dairy increases, so does fracture risk.

Low-Acid Eating

We need a theory that actually explains what causes fractures and how to prevent them. We need a theory that *works.*

The beginnings of just such a theory have been around for a century. Studies dating back to the 1880s suggest a different approach to osteoporosis, one that has nothing to do with milk, dairy, and calcium. This alternative view was fully articulated for the first time in 1968 in an article in *The Lancet.* Its coauthors, Amnon Wachman, M.D., of the State University of New York, and Daniel S. Bernstein, M.D., of Johns Hopkins, argued that the conventional wisdom was not the answer—but that something else was. Low-acid eating.

Among osteoporosis researchers, their article caused a stir. Low-acid eating represented a radically different approach to bone vitality. It turned the conventional wisdom upside down. But it neatly explained world fracture epidemiology and why milk, dairy, and calcium don't work. Compared with the calcium theory, it made much more sense.

A few researchers became intrigued. By the mid-1970s a trickle of studies began to be published, most of them supporting low-acid eating. More researchers got interested. During the 1980s the trickle became a stream, and by the 1990s a broad river of reports emerged in favor of low-acid eating. Today many researchers consider low-acid eating and daily exercise the best, most cost-effective way to strengthen bone and reduce fractures. Unfortunately, none of them seemed interested in writing a book for the general public. We got tired of waiting.

The low-acid explanation of osteoporosis is not flawless. Like virtually every issue in nutrition, questions remain. But compared with milk, dairy, calcium, and vitamin D, low-acid eating neatly explains who suffers osteoporotic fractures and why.

Evidence Recap

- All four studies of hip fracture rates worldwide show that they cluster in the countries that consume the most milk, dairy foods, and calcium. Countries with low milk and dairy intake generally have lower fracture rates.
- Only twenty-four of eight-six studies (28 percent) show that milk, dairy foods, and calcium pills by themselves or in combination prevent fractures. Sixty-two (72 percent) show that they do not.
- Only six of thirteen studies (46 percent) show that milk and dairy foods during childhood prevent fractures at any age. Seven trials (54 percent) show that milk and dairy during childhood make no difference to lifetime fracture risk.
- Seventeen of thirty-seven studies (46 percent) show that calcium and/or vitamin D prevent fractures. Twenty trials (54 percent) show no clear benefit. If calcium and vitamin D work, they would appear to reduce fracture risk about 17 percent. But many countries around the world have substantially lower fracture rates—without using calcium or vitamin D.
- Bottom line: Of the 140 fracture studies, forty-seven (34 percent) support the calcium theory. Ninety-three (66 percent) show no benefit. The evidence runs two to one against milk, dairy, and calcium.

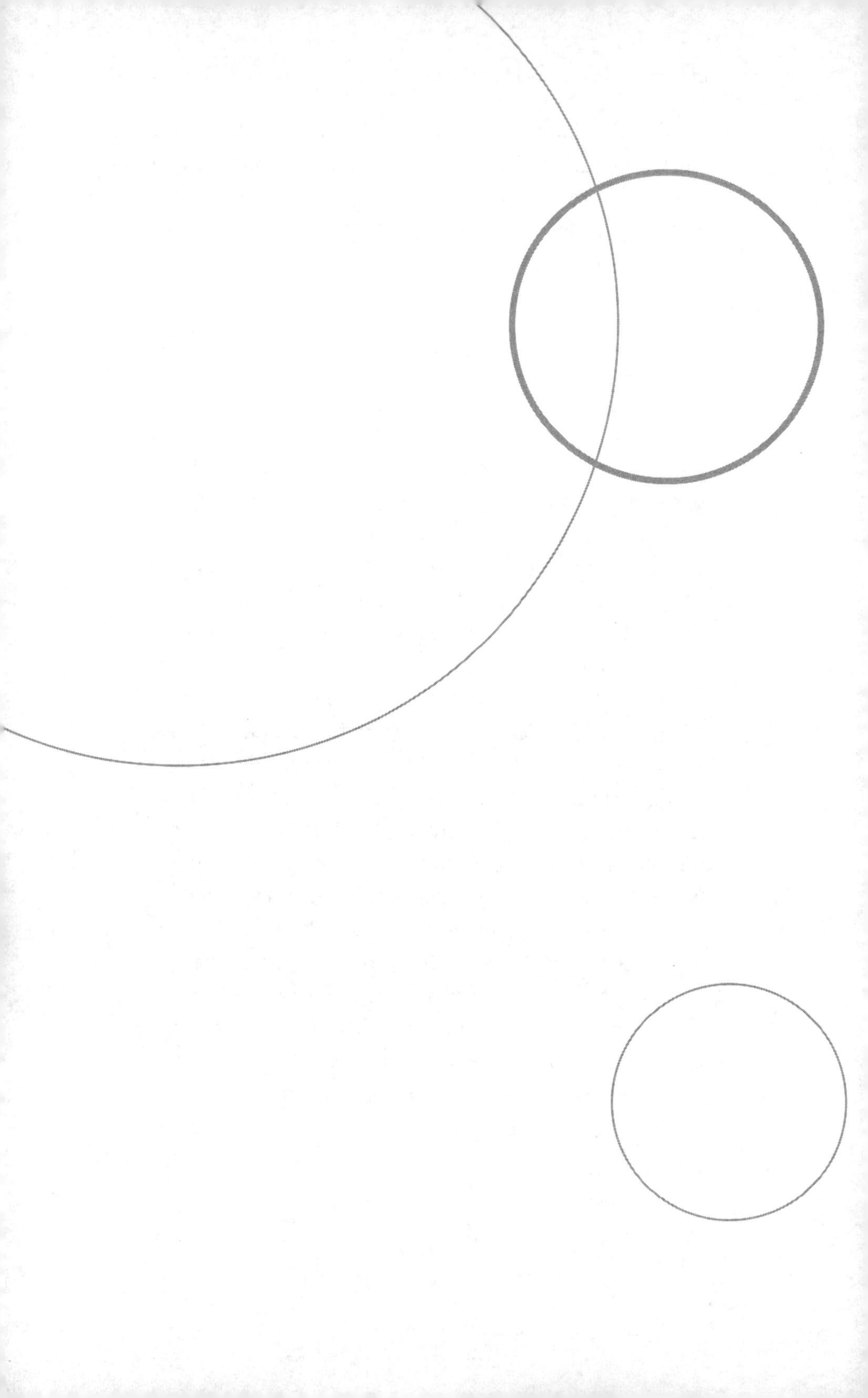

PART 2

The Bone Vitality Prescription: Low-Acid Eating and Daily Walking

The Key to Strong Bones and Fracture Prevention: The Bloodstream's Acid/Alkaline Balance

STRANGE AS THIS may sound, bone strength begins in the bloodstream. The blood is much more than the red stuff that conjures visions of Band-Aids. It's one of the most complex tissues in the body. Among its many functions, the blood:

- Transports oxygen to every cell to fuel all physiological processes
- Transports dozens of nutrients to nourish every cell
- Helps keep cells hydrated adequately
- Collects metabolic wastes and delivers them to the lungs, kidneys, liver, and digestive tract for elimination
- Carries the many hormones that influence everything from metabolism to energy to reproduction
- Provides a path for the cells and proteins of the immune system that defend the body against illness
- Plays a key role in the body's self-repair mechanisms, delivering the building blocks of new cells where they are needed

With so many vital responsibilities, the blood's composition is constantly changing as oxygen, nutrients, hormones, and other compounds enter it and as wastes, hormones, and other compounds depart. But at the same time, to function properly, the blood must maintain a very narrow chemical range. It's a delicate balancing act that makes the blood a marvel of self-regulation.

One crucial aspect of the blood's constant self-regulation is its pH, how acidic or alkaline it is. The letters *pH* stand for "potential of hydrogen." Hydrogen ions determine acidity. As hydrogen ions increase, the solution becomes more acidic. The pH scale ranges from 0 to 14. A neutral solution—neither acidic nor alkaline (basic)—has a pH of 7. A pH below 7 means the solution is acidic. A pH above 7 is alkaline.

Blood is slightly alkaline. Its normal pH varies from 7.35 to 7.45. If the blood's pH falls below 7.35 or rises above 7.45, the body cannot function properly. As a result, the body expends considerable energy to keep the blood's pH within its normal range.

When the Blood's pH Falls Below Normal

Have you ever taken Tums for acid indigestion? Tums is an antacid. Its main ingredient is calcium carbonate, which is highly alkaline. The calcium carbonate reacts with stomach acid. The carbonate neutralizes the acid, releasing calcium, which gets incorporated into urine. Calcium compounds play the same acid-neutralizing role in the blood.

Bone contains three calcium compounds: calcium carbonate, phosphate, and hydroxide. When the blood's pH falls below normal, the body *must* restore it as quickly as possible. It does this by pulling calcium compounds into the blood to neutralize excess acids. The body obtains these acid-neutralizing calcium compounds from the reservoir that contains 99 percent of the body's calcium store—bone.

What makes the blood acidic? Predominantly protein.

Proteins are combinations of 20 amino acids. Digestion breaks proteins into their component amino acids and sends them into the bloodstream. The more protein in the diet, the more amino acids enter the bloodstream. A high-protein diet reduces the blood's pH. It may or may not fall below 7.35, the lower end of its normal range. But even at the low end of normal, the body takes steps to raise the blood's pH—by drawing calcium compounds out of bone. This process is complex and involves special bone-dissolving cells called *osteoclasts*. (See sidebar on page 76.) But in simplest terms, a high-protein diet drops the blood's pH. To restore optimal pH, the body draws calcium compounds from bone.

Flushing Your Bones Down the Toilet

Calcium compounds pulled into the bloodstream quickly neutralize the flood of amino acids from digested protein. In the process, more calcium is drawn into the blood than is optimal. The kidneys filter this excess calcium from the blood, returning some of it to the bloodstream as needed and incorporating the rest into urine.

As the amount of protein in the diet increases, so does the amount of calcium excreted in urine. This is scientifically well established. According to the National Academy of Sciences, "1 gram of dietary protein increases urinary calcium excretion by 1 to 1.5 mg." One to 1.5 milligrams may not sound like much. But a four-ounce serving of chicken or beef contains about twenty grams of protein. Eat a chicken breast or a hamburger and you lose twenty to thirty milligrams of calcium. Over a lifetime, if that calcium is not returned to the bones, the loss can add up to a good deal of the skeleton—and eventually osteoporotic fractures.

Many studies demonstrate the link between dietary protein and calcium in urine:

- Harvard researchers analyzed the diets of premenopausal women and found that they consumed 1.1 grams of protein per kilogram (2.2 pounds) of weight, or three ounces a day for a woman weighing 140 pounds. The scientists also measured the women's urinary calcium and biochemical markers for bone loss. They then fed the women a diet containing the same number of calories they ordinarily ate, but with protein reduced to the amount recommended in U.S. dietary guidelines (0.8 gram per kilogram), about 1.8 ounces a day for a 140-pound woman. After two weeks on the lower-protein diet, "mean urinary calcium decreased 32 percent, and bone loss decreased 17 percent."

- University of Chicago researchers measured urinary calcium levels of healthy adults and then fed them a high-protein diet for four weeks. Their urinary calcium excretion increased 61 percent.
- In Detroit, Wayne State University researchers measured the urinary calcium output of healthy adults fed a diet containing 50 grams (1.8 ounces) of protein. When they then fed the group 150 grams (5.4 ounces) of protein, "the increase in protein intake doubled urinary calcium."
- Toronto researchers fed adults two different diets containing the same number of calories for one month each. In one, protein accounted for 16 percent of calories; in the other, 27 percent. On the high-protein diet, participants' daily urinary calcium output increased 63 percent.
- Finally, University of Rochester researchers measured adults' urinary calcium and then fed them a high-protein diet for forty days. On this diet urinary calcium increased 58 percent and the high-protein diet "depleted skeletal stores of calcium."

In addition to pulling calcium out of the blood, the kidneys process excess amino acids into ammonia, which is acidic and toxic to the central nervous system. The liver quickly converts ammonia into urea, also acidic, and incorporates it into urine, increasing urinary acidity. In the University of Chicago study just mentioned, in addition to measuring urinary calcium, the researchers measured urinary acidity. As participants' dietary protein increased, so did their urinary acidity.

Animal vs. Vegetable: Calcium Loss from Bone Differs by Type of Protein

From carrots to filet mignon, broccoli to cheese, cereals to chicken and fish, the vast majority of foods contain protein. As a result, most foods introduce amino acids into the bloodstream, increasing its acidity and the acidity of urine.

Table 7.1 charts the amount of acid various foods add to urine—and, by extension, to blood. Some foods acidify the urine considerably more than others. Compared with fruits and vegetables, animal foods—red meats, poultry, fish, eggs, and dairy items—introduce much more acid into urine and, therefore, into blood, causing greater loss of calcium compounds from bone. Grains, breads, and pastas also acidify the urine and blood, but less than most animal foods.

TABLE 7.1 The Effect of Common Foods on the Acidity of Urine

In addition to adding calcium to urine, a high-protein diet also makes urine more acidic. This table shows how common foods affect urinary acidity, expressed in milliequivalents (mEq), a standard chemical measure. Positive numbers indicate that the food makes urine acidic. As the number increases, so does urinary acidity. Negative numbers indicate that the food makes urine alkaline. As the numbers decrease, urine becomes more alkaline.

Food Item	Protein	Effect on Urine
(approx 4-oz. serving)	(grams)	(using standard scientific measures + numbers = acidic, − numbers = alkaline)
FRUITS AND JUICES		
Apple juice	0.1	–2.2
Apples	0.4	–2.2
Apricots	0.9	–4.8
Apricots, dried	3.4	–21.7
Avocados	2.0	–8.2
Bananas	1.2	–5.5
Cherries	0.9	–3.6
Figs, dried	3.3	–14.0
Grape juice	0.3	–1.0
Kiwi	1.1	–4.1
Lemon juice	0.3	–2.5
Orange juice	0.5	–2.9

continued

TABLE 7.1 The Effect of Common Foods on the Acidity of Urine (continued)

Food Item	Protein	Effect on Urine
(approx 4-oz. serving)	(grams)	(using standard scientific measures + numbers = acidic, − numbers = alkaline)
FRUITS AND JUICES (continued)		
Oranges	1.1	−2.7
Peaches	1.0	−2.4
Pears	0.3	−2.9
Pineapple	0.4	−2.7
Plums, dried (prunes)	2.2	−13.4
Raisins	2.1	−21.0
Strawberries	0.8	−2.2
Watermelon	0.5	−1.9
VEGETABLES		
Artichokes, boiled	2.9	−4.7
Asparagus	2.9	−0.4
Broccoli	4.4	−1.2
Cabbage	1.2	−4.7
Carrots	0.7	−4.9
Cauliflower	3.6	−4.0
Celery	0.5	−5.2
Chard, cooked	1.9	−12.4
Corn (sweet)	3.2	−1.8
Cucumber	0.7	−0.8
Eggplant	0.9	−3.4
Kale	3.3	−8.3
Leeks	1.6	−1.8
Lettuce (leaf)	0.8	−2.5
Lettuce (iceberg)	0.7	−1.6
Mushrooms (white)	1.8	−1.4
Mushrooms (portobello)	4.3	−3.7

TABLE 7.1 The Effect of Common Foods on the Acidity of Urine (continued)

Food Item	Protein	Effect on Urine
(approx 4-oz. serving)	(grams)	(using standard scientific measures + numbers = acidic, – numbers = alkaline)
VEGETABLES (continued)		
Onions	1.2	–1.5
Pepper (green)	0.8	–1.4
Pepper (red)	1.0	–3.4
Potatoes (russet)	2.1	–4.0
Potatoes (red with skin)	2.3	–7.1
Radish	0.7	–3.7
Snap peas	2.8	–2.0
Spinach	2.8	–14.0
Sweet potato (baked with skin)	2.0	–8.2
Tomato juice	0.8	–2.8
Tomatoes	0.7	–3.1
Zucchini	1.8	–4.6
BEANS		
Baked beans, canned, vegetarian	4.8	–0.8
Black beans, cooked	8.2	–1.5
Chickpeas (garbanzo)	8.9	2.6
Green beans	1.9	–3.1
Kidney beans	8.7	–0.7
Lentils (green and brown)	24.3	3.5
Peas	6.9	1.2
Pinto beans, cooked	9.0	–1.2
Soybeans, cooked	16.6	2.8
Soybeans, green (edamame)	16.6	–2.9
Tempeh, cooked	18.2	6.6

continued

TABLE 7.1 The Effect of Common Foods on the Acidity of Urine (continued)

Food Item	Protein	Effect on Urine
(approx 4-oz. serving)	(grams)	(using standard scientific measures + numbers = acidic, − numbers = alkaline)
BEANS (continued)		
Tofu, firm	8.2	−0.3
Veggie burger (soy-based)	15.7	5.1
NUTS		
Cashews	18.2	6.4
Coconut (raw)	3.3	−2.7
Hazelnuts	14.1	−2.8
Peanuts	25.6	8.3
Pecans	9.2	2.2
Pistachios	21.4	2.0
Walnuts	14.7	6.8
BEVERAGES		
Beer	0.3	−0.2
Coca-Cola	0.0	0.4
Cocoa (low-fat milk)	3.5	−0.4
Coffee	0.2	−1.4
Mineral water	0.0	−0.1
Red wine	0.2	−2.4
Soy milk, with calcium	2.9	0.0
Tea	0.1	−0.3
White wine	0.1	−1.2
FLESH FOODS		
Beef (lean)	20.3	7.8
Chicken (no skin)	20.5	8.7
Cod	17.4	7.1
Corned beef	26.9	13.2

TABLE 7.1 The Effect of Common Foods on the Acidity of Urine (continued)

Food Item	**Protein**	**Effect on Urine**
(approx 4-oz. serving)	(grams)	(using standard scientific measures + numbers = acidic, − numbers = alkaline)
FLESH FOODS (continued)		
Haddock	16.8	6.8
Herring	16.8	7.0
Hot dogs	9.5	6.7
Pork (lean)	20.7	7.9
Salami	19.3	11.6
Trout	23.5	10.8
Turkey (no skin)	21.9	9.9
Veal	21.1	9.0
CHEESE		
American (processed)	20.8	28.7
Camembert	20.9	14.6
Cheddar	31.5	26.4
Cheese (average of several)	24.7	19.2
Cottage	13.8	8.7
Gouda	24.0	18.6
Parmesan	39.4	34.2
MILK AND OTHER DAIRY FOODS		
Buttermilk	3.5	0.5
Cream (fresh, sour)	2.9	1.2
Ice cream (vanilla)	3.6	0.6
Milk (whole, evaporated)	8.4	1.1
Milk (whole)	3.2	0.7
Yogurt (whole milk, fruit)	5.1	1.2
Yogurt (whole milk, plain)	5.7	1.5

continued

TABLE 7.1 The Effect of Common Foods on the Acidity of Urine (continued)

Food Item	Protein	Effect on Urine
(approx 4-oz. serving)	(grams)	(using standard scientific measures + numbers = acidic, − numbers = alkaline)
EGGS		
Eggs (whole)	12.5	8.2
Egg whites	9.0	1.1
Egg yolks	16.1	23.4
GRAINS		
Bread, mixed flours	6.2	3.8
Bread, rye	6.8	4.1
Bread, white	7.0	1.8
Bread, whole wheat	7.0	1.8
Cornflakes	7.9	6.0
Crackers (rye)	9.4	3.3
Egg noodles	12.1	16.4
Flour, white	9.4	6.9
Flour, whole wheat	12.7	8.2
Oats (rolled, dry)	12.5	10.7
Quinoa, cooked	4.4	0.2
Rice, brown (dry)	6.7	12.5
Rice, white (dry)	7.3	4.6
Spaghetti, white	12.0	6.5
Spaghetti, whole wheat	13.4	7.3

Note 1: Dried fruits are the most alkaline plant foods, and cheeses, particularly hard cheeses, are the most acid-forming animal foods. The reason is that both are dehydrated. The water in fruit and milk dilutes the protein and alkaline material. Remove much of the water to make dried fruit or cheese, and either the alkaline material or the protein becomes more concentrated.

Note 2: Some foods that *seem* acidic make the urine (and blood) more alkaline. For example, oranges are rich in vitamin C, ascorbic acid. But as oranges are metabolized, their net effect is alkaline (−2.7).

SOURCES: Remer, T., and F. Manz. "Potential Renal Acid Loads of Foods and Its Influence on Urine pH," *Journal of the American Dietetic Association* (1995) 95: 791. And http://www.goutpal.com/potential-renal-acid-load.html.

With regard to osteoporotic fractures, animal foods are the main issue. Compared with fruits and vegetables, animal foods increase blood acidity much more—for two reasons:

- **Animal foods contain the most protein.** See Table 7.1. One serving of beef, chicken, turkey, pork, and many cheeses contains 15 grams of protein or more. In contrast, one serving of grain products averages 9 grams, and a typical serving of fruits and vegetables contains fewer than 2 grams. As a result, animal foods pump the most amino acids into the bloodstream—and force the body to draw the most calcium compounds from bone.

- **Animal foods are low in natural alkaline buffers.** Just as most foods contain protein, they also contain alkaline nutrients—calcium compounds and other minerals, notably potassium and magnesium. But like protein content, the alkaline content of foods varies considerably. Animal foods, especially cheeses and meats, don't contain much alkaline material. As animal foods get digested, their alkaline nutrients enter the bloodstream along with their amino acids and neutralize the blood's acidity to some extent. But compared with fruits and vegetables, animal foods are considerably higher in protein and lower in alkaline nutrients. Animal foods do not contain enough alkaline material to neutralize all the acids they introduce into the bloodstream. As a result, animal foods reduce the blood's pH. The body must draw calcium compounds from bone to restore optimal blood pH.

Fruits and vegetables are different—low in protein and high in alkaline nutrients. As fruits and vegetables get digested, only small amounts of amino acids enter the bloodstream, along with lots of alkaline nutrients. The alkaline material completely buffers the acids, and the body does not have to reach into bone for calcium compounds.

Dozens of studies show that, compared with fruits and vegetables, animal foods add more calcium to urine and cause more bone loss. Some of the studies:

- University of Texas researchers placed fifteen healthy young people on one of three diets containing progressively more animal protein: strict vegetarian (no animal foods), semi-vegetarian (dairy and eggs), or omnivorous (meats). Subjects average urinary calcium ranged from 103 milligrams a day on the strict vegetarian diet to 150 milligrams a day on the omnivorous diet—46 percent higher.

- British researchers surveyed the diets of 14,563 adults and then measured their bone mineral density. Those who ate the most meat, fish, eggs, and grains and the fewest fruits and vegetables had the lowest BMD. As their fruit and vegetable consumption increased relative to animal foods, their BMD also increased.

- Japanese researchers surveyed the diets of 755 adults and compared their urinary calcium based on the type of protein they consumed. "The correlation of calcium excretion with animal protein was significantly positive in both sexes and in every age group. Excess protein may augment calcium excretion in urine."

- Cornell researchers surveyed the diets of 764 Chinese women and then measured the calcium and acid in their urine. "Urinary excretion of calcium and acids was positively associated with intakes of animal protein, but negatively with plant protein, because of the alkaline nature of plant foods."

- Finally, Harvard researchers surveyed the diets, lifestyles, and health of 85,900 nurses in 1980 and then followed them for twelve years. Consumption of "animal protein was associated with an increased risk of fracture. But no association was found for consumption of vegetable protein."

The Calcium Paradox Explained

In Part 1 we showed that the calcium theory does not explain fracture risk in the real world. The low-acid theory offers an elegant explanation.

Milk and dairy foods are high in animal protein but low in alkaline nutrients. They flood the bloodstream with amino acids but don't buffer them. To neutralize those acids, the body must draw calcium compounds from bone. As a result, we would not expect milk and dairy foods to prevent fractures—and they don't.

Of course, milk, dairy, and calcium supplements are high in calcium. Some of the mineral becomes incorporated into bone. But not enough to really strengthen bone because it's being pulled out as it's going in. Calcium is out of balance. That's why two-thirds of clinical trials show that milk, dairy foods, and calcium supplements do not prevent fractures.

Why do countries consuming the most milk and dairy products have the highest fracture rates? Because these affluent Western countries also consume the most meat, poultry, and fish.

Meanwhile, compared with Western nations, the countries whose populations consume the least milk and dairy also consume less total animal protein—less meat and more fruits and vegetables. As a result, their diets build bone instead of destroying it.

Anthony Sebastian, M.D., professor emeritus of nephrology at the University of California, San Francisco (UCSF), led the research team that published the 2000 survey of worldwide fracture rates. His group correlated fractures to all the countries' consumption of animal and plant protein (Figure 7.1). The dots look scattered, but when analyzed using standard statistical techniques, they form a straight line. As intake of animal protein rises, so does the rate of hip fracture. The straight-line relationship is a hallmark of a causal "dose-response relationship." As animal protein consumption increases, the hip fracture rate rises steadily, as we would expect if the former caused the latter.

Figure 7.2 shows that as intake of vegetable protein rises, the rate of hip fracture falls. Here again, we see a dose-response relationship.

Finally, Figure 7.3 shows that as the ratio of vegetable-to-animal protein increases, the hip fracture rate plummets.

In the figures, the term *person-years* combines the number of persons and the number of years they were followed.

FIGURE 7.1 Hip Fractures and Animal Protein Intake

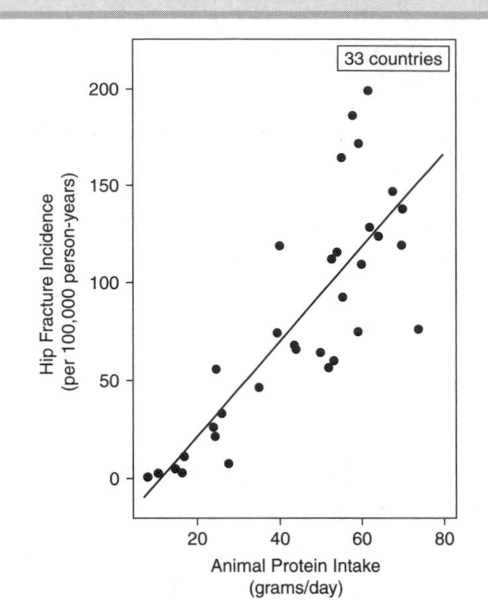

As animal protein intake increases, so does the rate of hip fracture. Results are highly statistically significant: p = < 0.001.

FIGURE 7.2 Hip Fractures and Vegetable Protein Intake

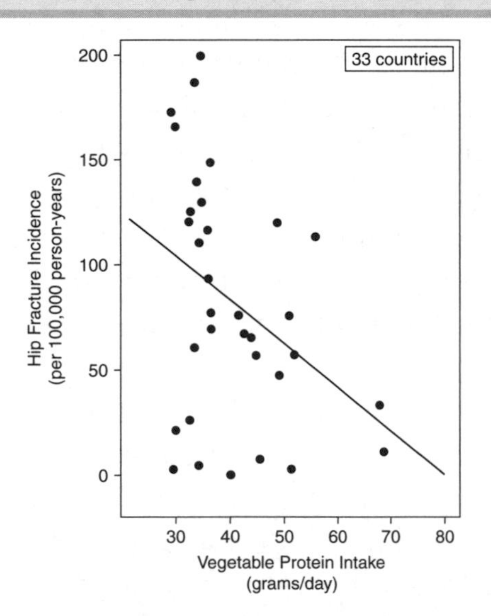

As consumption of protein from fruits and vegetables rises, the rate of hip fracture falls. Results are statistically significant: p = < 0.04.

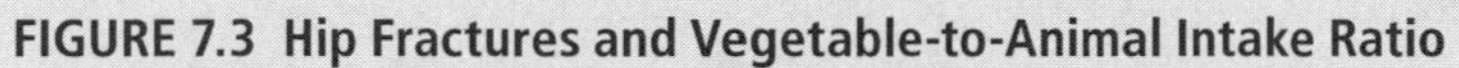

FIGURE 7.3 Hip Fractures and Vegetable-to-Animal Intake Ratio

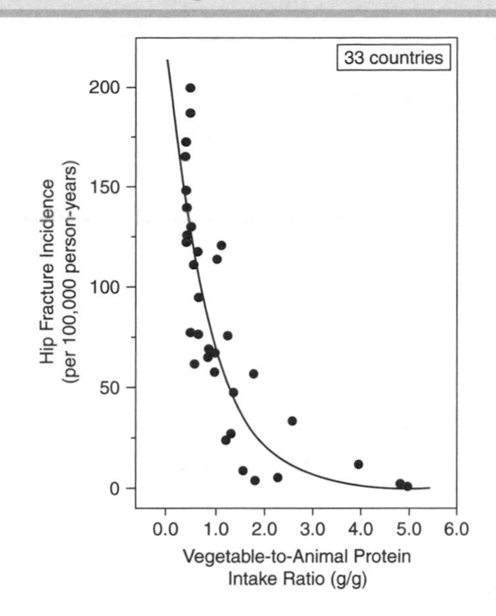

As we move to the right on the horizontal axis—from 0 to 6.0—the populations studied consume more vegetable protein relative to animal protein, up to six times as much. More vegetable protein relative to animal protein results in substantially reduced risk of hip fracture. Results are highly statistically significant: $p = < 0.001$.

The Sebastian team concludes: "The high incidence of hip fracture in industrialized countries is caused by the cumulative effects on bone of the body's chronic high net acid load. This high net acid load, in turn, is the result of disproportionate consumption of animal (acid) foods relative to vegetable (alkaline) foods. Otherwise healthy individuals who eat net acid-producing diets are in a chronic state of low-grade metabolic acidosis [acidic blood and urine]. The body adapts through dissolution of bone. Over decades, the magnitude of a daily positive acid balance [that is, chronically acidic blood and urine] may be sufficient to induce osteoporosis. Moderation of animal food consumption and an increased ratio of vegetable-to-animal food consumption may confer a fracture-protective effect."

Several other studies corroborate the Sebastian team's conclusion:

- The 1992 study of worldwide hip fracture rates also correlates fractures with consumption of animal protein (Figure 7.4). The researchers conclude: "Female hip fracture incidence is highest in industrialized countries. A possible explanation is that elevated metabolic acid production associated with a high-animal-protein diet might lead to chronic bone dissolution. When female fracture rates derived from thirty-four studies in sixteen countries were correlated with estimates of dietary animal protein, a strong, positive association was found."
- Other UCSF researchers—not the Sebastian group—surveyed the diets of 1,035 elderly women and then tracked them for seven years. As the ratio of animal to vegetable protein increased—that is, when the women ate lots of animal foods and not many plant foods—their risk of hip fracture soared. Compared with women eating the most plant-based diet, those who ate the most animal foods and the fewest fruits and vegetables suffered *3.7 times more hip fractures.*

FIGURE 7.4 Risk of Hip Fracture and Dietary Animal Consumption

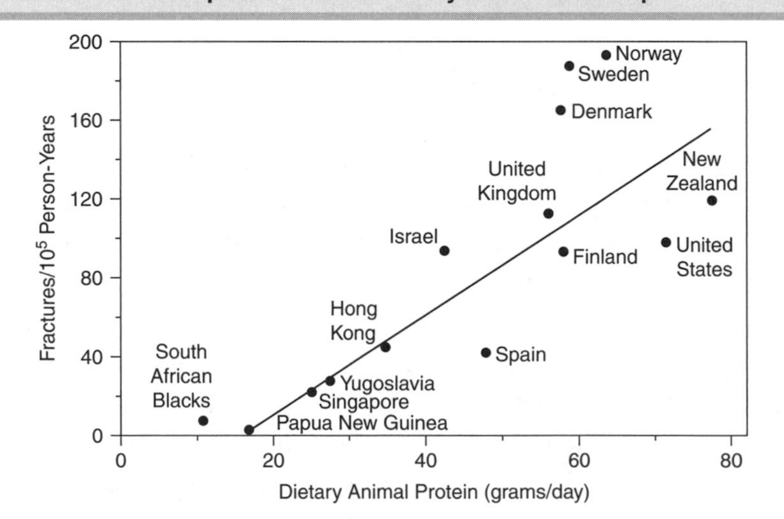

As dietary animal protein consumption increases, so does risk of hip fracture. Results are statistically significant: $p = 0.024$.

- Swedish researchers surveyed the protein intake of 39,787 adults and followed them for eleven years. Intake of vegetable protein made no difference to the group's hip fracture risk. But as intake of animal protein increased, so did hip fracture risk. Compared with those who ate no animal foods, participants who consumed the most suffered *twice as many hip fractures.*
- Harvard researchers followed the diets and forearm fracture risk of 85,900 women nurses for twelve years. "Animal protein was associated with an increased risk of fracture. No association was found for consumption of vegetable protein."

Uriel S. Barzel, M.D., a professor of endocrinology at Albert Einstein College of Medicine in New York, and Linda K. Massey, Ph.D., a professor of nutrition at Washington State University in Spokane, summarize these findings this way: "The average American diet is high in animal protein and low in fruits and vegetables. This generates a large amount of acid. The kidneys respond with net acid excretion [in urine]. Concurrently, the skeleton supplies [calcium compounds as a] buffer resulting in resorption [loss] of bone. Different food proteins differ greatly in their acid load. A diet high in acid-producing proteins causes excessive calcium loss from bone. The addition of buffers such as fruits and vegetables results in less acidic urine, and less calciuria [calcium in urine]. Bone resorption may be halted, and bone accretion [building] may occur."

Calcium Balance: Don't Just Open the Faucet; Plug the Drain

Imagine a bathtub filled with enough water to take a luxurious bath. The tub's faucet can't be turned off, but inflow can be regulated from a trickle to a flood. The tub also has a drain that cannot be plugged, but outflow can also be regulated from a little to a lot. How can you keep the water level where you want it? Obviously, match the inflow and outflow.

Calcium in bone works the same way. What you eat represents the inflow—how much of the mineral is available to build bone. What you eat also governs outflow—how much of the mineral you flush away in urine.

The calcium theory focuses only on the inflow. Our health authorities tell us to consume more, MORE, *MORE* calcium—1,000 milligrams a day for adults aged nineteen to fifty and 1,200 milligrams a day for those fifty-one and older. Yet the United States has an epidemic of osteoporosis.

Our health authorities seem blind to the effect of the outflow. The typical American diet—high in meat and dairy foods—draws a great deal of calcium compounds from bone, more of the mineral than eating and calcium supplements replace. Hence our fracture epidemic.

People in many countries around the world consume only five hundred milligrams of calcium a day, half of what American health authorities recommend, or less, yet have fracture rates only a small fraction of ours. Not as much calcium flows in through the faucet, but even less drains away.

It's all about *calcium balance*. That's the term researchers use to describe the coordination of the faucet and the drain, the inflow and outflow. It doesn't matter how much calcium you gobble down if you're flushing more away in urine. With low-acid eating—lots of fruits and vegetables, a moderate amount of grain products, and little, if any, meat, poultry, fish, and dairy—you keep the faucet more open than the drain. Calcium comes in, so you build bone. But very little goes out, so you don't lose it.

Milk and Dairy Are Not Necessary: You CAN Get Enough Calcium for Strong Bones Entirely from Plant Foods

Many Americans believe that it's simply not possible to get enough calcium for strong bones without milk and dairy foods. Not so.

About one-third of the typical American's calcium intake comes from nondairy sources: fruits, vegetables, grains, beans, nuts, seeds, eggs, and animal foods. In addition, less than a third of the calcium in milk and dairy foods is actually absorbed into the bloodstream. Finally, dairy foods—even milk fortified with vitamin D—lack the many other nutrients necessary to build strong bones. (See Chapter 9.)

Meanwhile, few Americans appreciate how much calcium can be obtained from fruits and vegetables. (See Table 7.2.) Compared with calcium from dairy foods, as much—or more—of the calcium in many fruits and vegetables enters the bloodstream. In particular, about one-half to two-thirds of the calcium in dark green leafy veg-

TABLE 7.2 Plant Sources of Calcium

Note: While U.S. health authorities recommend calcium intake of 1,000 mg/day, residents of many countries around the world have substantially lower fracture rates than Americans while consuming less than 500 mg of calcium per day.

Source of Calcium	mg Calcium
Tofu, firm, 1 cup	506
Soy milk, calcium-fortified, 1 cup	368
Collard greens, cooked, 1 cup	356
Spinach, cooked from frozen, 1 cup	292
Figs, 10 dried	269
Soybeans, cooked, 1 cup	260
Turnip greens, cooked from frozen, 1 cup	248
Fortified ready-to-eat cereals (Total, etc.), 1 oz.	236 to 1,043
White beans, canned, 1 cup	192
Kale, cooked from frozen, 1 cup	180
Okra, cooked from frozen, 1 cup	176
Molasses, blackstrap, 1 tbsp	172
Beet greens, cooked from frozen, 1 cup	164
Bok choy, Chinese cabbage, cooked from fresh, 1 cup	158
Dandelion greens, cooked from fresh, 1 cup	148
Almonds, dry roasted, 1 oz.	80
Raisins, ⅔ cup	53

SOURCE: Agricultural Research Service, U.S. Dept. of Agriculture

TABLE 7.3 Foods Rich in Calcium: Amount Needed to Absorb Approximately 100 mg Calcium

Notice that compared with animal foods, plant foods contain less calcium per serving. However, the body absorbs more calcium from plant foods than from dairy foods. As a result, the actual amount of plant foods required to absorb the same amount of calcium is lower than one might think.

Food	Standard Serving Size	Calcium/ Standard Serving	Calcium Absorbed/ Serving*	Amount Needed to Absorb Approx. 100 mg Calcium
Total Plus cereal	¾ cup	1,000	301	⅓ cup
Low-fat yogurt	8 oz.	400	128	¾ cup
Orange juice, calcium-fortified	1 cup	300	108	⅞ cup
2% milk	1 cup	297	95	1 cup
Soy milk, calcium-fortified	1 cup	300	93	1 cup
Basic Four cereal	1 cup	306	92	1 cup heaping
Cheddar cheese	1 oz.	204	66	1½ oz.
Mozzarella cheese, part skim	1 oz.	183	59	1¾ oz.
Sesame seeds, unhulled	1 oz.	280	58	1¾ oz.
Firm tofu, calcium-set	3 oz.	172	53	⅔ cup
Kale, frozen	½ cup	90	53	1 cup
Turnip greens, frozen	½ cup	99	51	1 cup
Mustard greens, frozen	½ cup	76	44	1⅛ cups
Chinese cabbage, bok choy, boiled	½ cup	79	43	1⅛ cups
White beans, cooked	1 cup	161	35	2¾ cups
Broccoli, frozen	½ cup	47	29	1⅔ cups
Brussels sprouts, boiled	½ cup	28	18	2¾ cups
Spinach, boiled	½ cup	122	6	8 cups

* Calculations by AJL based on USDA data and published on calcium absorption.

etables (spinach, chard, kale, etc.) gets absorbed. (See Table 7.3.) In addition, plant foods are alkaline, so they don't force the body to draw calcium compounds from bone. And plant foods also contain the other nutrients necessary to build bone.

The proof is in the epidemiology. As we've seen, residents of countries that consume the most dairy products have the highest fracture rates. For residents of countries that consume little or no dairy, but lots of plant foods, osteoporosis is not much of a problem. They get enough calcium for strong bones from plant foods.

Finally, several studies have asked how much calcium American vegans consume. Vegans are the strictest vegetarians. They eat only plant foods (fruits, vegetables, grains, legumes, nuts, and seeds), no meats, poultry, fish, milk, dairy items, or eggs. Researchers at Penn State calculate that the typical vegan consumes around 620 milligrams of calcium per day. This is 40 to 50 percent below what U.S. health authorities recommend. But it's *more* than most Asians consume—and as we've seen, they are at very low risk for osteoporotic fractures. You don't need 1,000 milligrams of calcium a day if you don't flush your bones away in urine. Five hundred milligrams a day is just fine. After reviewing all of the studies on calcium and bone health, the World Health Association came to the same conclusion—that 500 milligrams of calcium per day is recommended for adults in countries with high osteoporosis risk like the United States. It's not difficult to consume that much—or more—from plant foods.

To Save Your Bones, Eat a Low-Acid Diet

Vegan eating is likely best for bone vitality—assuming that the vegan diet contains lots of fruits, vegetables, and legumes and only moderate amounts of mildly acid-forming cereals, breads, and pastas. A diet based on fruits and vegetables, with some legumes and grains, contains more than enough calcium for strong bones and more than enough protein for good health. The recommended intake for protein is 0.8 grams per kilogram body weight for most adults according to the American Dietetic Association and other health authorities. This works out for most people to about 10 percent of total calories consumed. Currently, most omnivorous Americans consume at least twice this amount putting bones at risk. A vegan, vegetarian, or other low-acid diet will help to moderate protein intake to recommended levels. The protein in fruits and vegetables comes with a great deal of alkaline buffering material, so the body does not have to reach into bone for calcium compounds. Finally, plant foods also contain the many noncalcium nutrients essential for building strong bones, nutrients often deficient in diets based on animal foods.

A vegan diet is also best for health in general:

- In a series of landmark studies over the past twenty-five years, Dean Ornish, M.D., has demonstrated that a near-vegan diet combined with daily walking, yoga, meditation, and a support group can actually *reverse* heart disease. The Ornish program opens clogged arteries without drugs or surgery, a feat no medical treatment can match.
- Caldwell Esselstyn, M.D., of the Cleveland Clinic observed reversal of heart disease with a vegan diet paired with cholesterol-lowering medication.
- Neal Barnard, M.D., and colleagues at the Washington, DC, Center for Clinical Research have shown that a vegan diet is an effective way to lose weight and reverse diabetes.
- Dean Ornish has also shown that a vegan diet slows the progression of prostate cancer.

Not everyone is ready to choose a vegan diet. The good news for those who are not is that to enjoy strong bones and a low risk of fractures, there's no need to completely swear off meat, poultry, fish, eggs, milk, cheese, yogurt, pizza, and ice cream. Instead, eat a low-acid diet—only small portions of acid-generating foods—while simultaneously consuming lots of fruits and vegetables. (See Chapter 11 for tips on low-acid eating.)

Lots of fruits and vegetables and little or no meat. We're not the only ones advocating this. Many major health and medical organizations make the same recommendations: the National Cancer Institute, the American Heart Association, the American Dietetic Association, and the Centers for Disease Control and Prevention (CDC). They all endorse a plant-based, low-acid diet that includes at least five servings of fruits and vegetables a day and preferably six to ten, with less meat (several meat-free days every week), fewer high-fat dairy products, and less fast food and junk food.

This approach to eating goes by several names: *vegetarian, Asian style, Mediterranean*. We call it *low-acid eating*. Whatever you call it, a diet that includes at least five daily servings of fruits and vegetables, moderate amounts of grain products, and low intake of animal foods is the healthiest nonvegan way to eat. In addition to improving bone health, many studies show that Mediterranean eating and other low-acid diets also reduce risk of heart disease, cancer, Alzheimer's disease, and many other chronic conditions.

Returning to bone health, let's consider four meals: (1) a cheeseburger and french fries, (2) a chicken sandwich on whole wheat bread with green beans, (3) spaghetti with a tomato-vegetable sauce and a fruit salad, and (4) vegetable brochettes with rice and a green salad with walnuts. Using the information from Table 7.1, it's easy to see how the typical American meat-and-potatoes meal harms bone and how a low-acid meal with little or no meat and dairy strengthens it:

Food	**Acidic (+ figures) or Alkaline (− figures)**
Hamburger patty (4 oz.)	7.8
Bun, white (2 oz., 3.7 ÷ 2)	1.85
Cheese (1 oz., 19.2 ÷ 4)	4.2
Potatoes (4 oz.)	−4.0
Total	**9.85 (acidic; hurts bone)**
Chicken breast (4 oz.)	8.7
Whole wheat bread (2 oz., 1.8 ÷ 2)	0.9
Green beans (4 oz.)	−3.1
Total	**6.5 (acidic; hurts bone)**
Spaghetti (4 oz.)	6.5
Tomato sauce (4 oz.)	−2.8
Mixed vegetables (4 oz.)	−4.0
Parmesan cheese (0.25 oz., 34.2 ÷ 16)	2.14
Mixed fruit (4 oz.)	−3.0
Total	**−1.16 (alkaline; helps bone)**

Food	**Acidic (+ figures) or Alkaline (− figures)**
Vegetable brochettes: mushrooms, zucchini, tomatoes, onions (8 oz. total)	−5.5
Pineapple for brochettes (2 oz.)	−1.4
Rice (2 oz. dry)	2.3
Lettuce (4 oz.)	−2.5
Cucumber (2 oz.)	−0.4
Orange (2 oz.)	−1.3
Walnuts (1 oz.)	1.7
Total	**−7.1 (alkaline; helps bone)**

Duke researchers demonstrated the bone benefits of low-acid eating from a perspective that, ironically, had nothing to do with osteoporosis. Their study was an offshoot of the DASH program, Dietary Approaches to Stop Hypertension, a large, ongoing research effort aimed at controlling high blood pressure without drugs, using just a plant-based, low-acid diet. Since the mid-1990s, many DASH studies have shown that this diet does, indeed, reduce blood pressure. Meanwhile, as evidence mounted that low-acid eating also reduces osteoporosis risk, the Duke researchers placed 186 adults on either a typical American diet or the DASH diet. A month later, those eating the burger-and-fries diet showed bone loss. The people on the DASH diet showed the opposite, stronger bones and bone building.

The Osteoporosis Cure

We'll say it again: The calcium theory does not explain worldwide fracture rates. And by a margin of two to one, milk, dairy foods, and calcium pills (even with added vitamin D) fail to prevent fractures.

The low-acid theory explains much more. Despite the world's highest intake of milk, dairy foods, and calcium supplements, Western countries have an osteoporosis epidemic because they eat so much blood-acidifying animal protein and not enough alkaline fruits and vegetables. This mix produces a net outflow of calcium from bone—and eventually fractures.

Back in 1968, in the article that first suggested low-acid eating as the osteoporosis cure, Amnon Wachman and Daniel Bernstein noted: "Diets in the West usually include a large amount of meat. The urine of [those eating a meat-based diet] is acidic. The association between this observation and the increasing incidence of bone loss with age is inescapable. Increased incidence of osteoporosis with age may represent the result of life-long use of the buffering capacity of the calcium in bone [to maintain normal blood pH]. It might be worthwhile to consider decreasing the rate of bone loss with a diet favoring alkaline [urine]. This diet would emphasize ingestion of fruits and vegetables."

And it's not just to the benefit of our bones that we boost fruits and vegetables in our diets and limit animal foods. In a 2001 article in the *American Journal of Clinical Nutrition*, D. Mark Hegsted, Ph.D., a researcher with the Human Nutrition Center of the U.S. Department of Agriculture in Washington, explained:

> Although high-calcium intakes have long been recommended to prevent osteoporosis, there is little evidence that milk, dairy foods, and calcium supplements prevent fractures. Longstanding U.S. recommendations to increase calcium intake have had little or no effect on the prevalence of osteoporosis or fractures. Today, recommended calcium intakes in the U.S. are so high that it is difficult, if not impossible, to devise a practical diet that provides that much.
>
> Worldwide data raise serious questions about the relation between calcium intake and fractures. A large proportion of the world's population consumes diets low in milk, dairy, and calcium, yet [their bone development is normal], and these populations do not have the excessive fracture rates [seen in the U.S.].
>
> Like coronary artery disease, osteoporotic fractures are largely a disease of Western societies. Around the world, rates of osteoporotic fracture are roughly correlated with the incidence of heart disease. Countries consuming a Western diet—primarily the United States, Canada, and Western Europe—have high rates of both heart disease and fractures, suggesting shared causal factors.

The osteoporosis cure involves eating two or more servings of fruits and vegetables at every meal, going easy on the breads, cereals, and pastas, and limiting animal foods to, at most, a few times a week. In addition to substantially reducing risk of osteoporosis and fractures, this diet also helps prevent heart disease, most cancers, and other serious conditions.

Calcium Compounds in Bone: How the Body Adds and Removes Them

When we see bones in museums, they look as dead as chalk. Living bone is very much alive. Like the skin and other tissues, it undergoes constant breakdown and renewal. In each of us at any given moment, there are one to ten million tiny spots where old bone is being dissolved and new bone is being created. Over a typical lifetime this process replaces the entire skeleton more than six times.

Bone is solid, but it's also elastic enough under normal circumstances to tolerate stretching, twisting, bending, and jumping without breaking. To accomplish this, bone is constructed around a spongy, elastic, honeycomb core, a protein-rich collagen matrix that accounts for about 20 percent of skeletal weight. Calcium compounds and the other bone minerals are packed into this matrix much the way stucco is applied to wire mesh. The collagen provides the framework and flexibility; the minerals, the rigidity and strength.

While typical daily activities don't cause fractures, as we walk, run, jump, twist, bend, and ascend and descend stairs, our bones suffer microscopic damage. The body recognizes these weak spots and quickly marshals its repair mechanisms.

Bone repair (remodeling) is similar to highway repair. But instead of road crews removing broken pavement and filling holes with new asphalt, the body dispatches special cells. The first to arrive are osteoclasts. They clear old bone. They secrete acid that dissolves damaged bone, creating a microcavity. When all the weak bone has been dissolved, the osteoclasts die.

Their deaths signal the body to send in other cells, osteoblasts, that fill the cavity and then draw calcium, magnesium, phosphorus, and other minerals from the blood to form crystals that bond to the collagen. Over a few months, the collagen and minerals harden into new bone and the osteoblasts become mature bone cells, alive but no longer mobile, locked into bone.

Microfractures are not the only events that stimulate osteoclast bone clearing. These cells also go into overdrive when the blood's pH drops below normal. In addition, low blood pH suppresses the bone-building osteoblasts. Bone building is important—but not as important as maintaining blood pH in the normal range. Meanwhile, alkaline blood suppresses bone-dissolving osteoclasts and stimulates bone-building osteoblasts.

Bottom line: Blood pH regulates the cells that build bone and draw calcium compounds from it. Optimally alkaline blood stimulates bone building. Blood pH below optimal levels simulates bone loss.

Mediterranean and Other Health-Enhancing Low-Acid Ways to Eat

The health benefits of Mediterranean eating were first documented by Ancel Keys, Ph.D. (1904–2004), a professor of physiology at the University of Minnesota. During World War II, Keys became intrigued by reports that heart disease rates plummeted in war-torn Europe in countries with meat and dairy shortages and then rose after the war as animal foods became more available. At that time scientists knew little about the connection between diet and heart disease. After the war Keys and his wife toured Europe and

continued

Africa, looking for clues that might explain the changes in European heart disease rates. They were among the first to connect heart disease risk with blood levels of a compound found only in animal foods, cholesterol.

Starting in the late 1950s, Keys launched one of the first large prospective trials, a twenty-year study of diet and heart disease involving twelve thousand middle-aged men in seven countries: Finland, Greece, Italy, Japan, the United States, and the former Yugoslavia. This study was among the first to link heart disease to a diet high in cholesterol and saturated (animal) fat.

But Keys's findings also contained a surprise. Japanese men consumed the least cholesterol and saturated fat—but did *not* have the lowest rate of heart disease. The men of Crete did. They ate almost as much total fat as the men with the most heart disease, the Finns, but their diet was very different. The Cretans ate some meat, poultry, and dairy, but much less than the Finns. Most of their dietary fat came from olive oil. The Cretans ate mostly fruits and vegetables, plus moderate amounts of beans and whole grains.

Keys and others showed that, like the Cretans, the populations of other Mediterranean countries—Spain, Italy, and Greece—consumed almost as much total fat as Americans at that time but had much lower rates of heart disease. They also ate lots of fruits and vegetables, beans, and whole grains and not much meat and dairy. This has become known as *Mediterranean eating*.

In addition to its bone-building benefits, more than a hundred studies document other benefits of low-acid, Mediterranean eating, chief among them reduced risk of heart disease and cancer:

- British researchers periodically surveyed the diets of 594,580 members of AARP (formerly the American Association of Retired Persons). After ten years, compared with those who ate a typical American diet (high in meats, low in fruits and vegetables), those who embraced Mediterranean eating had

21 percent fewer heart disease deaths and 14 percent fewer cancer deaths. "The results provide strong evidence for a beneficial effect of Mediterranean diet."

- You don't have to be elderly to benefit from Mediterranean eating. Greek researchers recruited 42,237 women under fifty and followed them for twelve years. Even in this relatively young group, Mediterranean eating cut deaths from all causes by 13 percent and cancer deaths by 16 percent.
- Other Greek researchers followed 74,607 men and women over age sixty for up to ten years. As commitment to Mediterranean eating increased, deaths from all causes decreased. "The plant-based diet is associated with lower all-cause mortality."
- A third team of Greek researchers tracked the diet and health of 74,607 men and women over age sixty in Denmark, France, Germany, Greece, Italy, the Netherlands, Spain, and Sweden. As a Mediterranean style of eating increased, deaths from heart disease and cancer decreased.
- Italian researchers urged 11,323 men and women who'd had heart attacks to adopt a Mediterranean diet. Six years later, most had shifted their diets toward Mediterranean eating, but some had not. Compared with those who maintained their old ways, those who went Mediterranean cut their risk of dying from all causes by 49 percent.
- At Columbia University, researchers tracked the diets and brain function of 2,258 elderly men and women. After four years, compared with those who ate the most animal protein, participants who ate a Mediterranean diet were 40 percent less likely to develop Alzheimer's disease.
- Finally, Spanish researchers reviewed forty-three studies of the effects of Mediterranean eating and consistently found significantly lower cholesterol, less high blood pressure and diabetes, and less risk of death from heart disease and cancer.

continued

However, Mediterranean eating is not the only low-acid diet that reduces risk of osteoporosis, heart disease, cancer, and other serious conditions. Starting in the 1980s, T. Colin Campbell, Ph.D., of Cornell and colleagues in China and in England launched a huge study of the effects of diet on risk of cancer and other diseases in 130 villages widely dispersed around rural China.

China was an ideal setting for three reasons: Rates of heart disease, cancer, and other conditions varied tremendously around rural China. At the time, rural Chinese tended to live in the same region all their lives. And rural Chinese tended to eat diets unique to their regions, ranging from almost entirely vegetarian to moderate amounts of meats and fish. In addition, on average, rural Chinese diets contained three times as many fruits and vegetables as the typical American diet and, at most, only one-third the animal foods, usually less.

The China Study came up with striking findings. Compared with Americans, rural Chinese had substantially lower rates of heart disease, many cancers (breast, colon, prostate), and osteoporosis. In addition, among the Chinese, those who consumed the fewest animal foods had the lowest rates of heart disease, cancer, and osteoporosis. The researchers concluded that to achieve a substantial reduction in chronic disease in the United States, Americans must make a substantial shift away from animal foods (meat, dairy, and eggs) to plant-based foods (fruits, vegetables, grains, and legumes). They also observed that the more the diet was tipped toward plant foods the better for reducing chronic disease—meaning that a diet with no animal foods is better than one that has some small amounts of animal foods on most days.

Note: True Mediterranean and Chinese diets are *much different* from what you find on the menus of Spanish, Italian, Greek, and Chinese restaurants in the United States. American restaurateurs have piled on the meat, poultry, fish, seafood, and cheese. Those eating traditional Mediterranean or Chinese diets eat animal foods only a few times a week with portions the size of a deck of cards or smaller. Several days a week they eat no animal foods, except perhaps a sprinkle of cheese on pasta dishes. They substitute beans or tofu for animal foods and base their diet on fruits and vegetables, plus grains and legumes.

Vegan, vegetarian, Mediterranean, and Chinese and other Asian diets are among the healthiest ways to eat. In addition to reducing risk of heart disease and cancer, they also prevent fractures.

The Acidifiers: Why Animal Foods? Why Grains?

Evolution is elegant. It has created millions of species marvelously adapted to their environmental niches. Many strange creatures thrive under hostile conditions: in the freezing arctic, in dark subterranean caverns, even in hot springs filled with boiling water.

In contrast, we humans seem poorly adapted to our niche. Many of the foods most of us take for granted—meat, dairy, fish, milk, eggs, bread, cereals, and pasta—harm us by acidifying our blood and causing osteoporosis. Why haven't we evolved as elegantly as other creatures?

Because how we produce food has changed must faster than we have evolved.

The first humanlike creatures, the great apes, appeared thirty million years ago. They subsisted on fruits, seeds, and nuts, along with some vegetables, and very occasionally meat found by scavenging.

Around seven million years ago the ape and protohuman lines diverged. Protohumans continued to eat a diet based on fruit, vegetables, seeds, and nuts, with only a little meat and no dairy after weaning. Like other mammals, after infancy, protohumans lost the ability to produce lactase, the enzyme that allows digestion of milk sugar (lactose). By today's standards, protohumans were primitive and brutish, but they were well adapted to their environment. More than twenty million years of evolution had genetically prepared them to thrive on the diet they ate.

By five million years ago protohumans had an estimated 99 percent of the genetic makeup we have today. "They did not have a problem with weak, fracture-prone bones," says Colorado State University professor Loren Cordain, Ph.D., an authority on the Paleolithic diet, "because they ate lots of fruits and vegetables, which provided enough calcium to build strong bones."

Two million years ago, the human line diverged from small apes (chimps). Humans evolved smaller stomachs and larger brains. More brain power led to the invention of the Paleolithic era's key tools—stone knives and spears. This advance made hunting easier. Suddenly meat assumed greater importance. But fruits, vegetables, seeds, and nuts continued to supply an estimated two-thirds of protohumans' calories. Try hunting with a stone spear. It's much easier to gather plants.

Fish bones and seafood shells first appeared at Paleolithic sites around 130,000 years ago. But they didn't become widespread until 20,000 years ago.

Agriculture emerged around ten thousand years ago in the Middle East, China, and the Americas. Within a few thousand years, grains became a human staple and most hunter-gatherers settled down to farm.

Agriculture brought the domestication of animals and better fishing technology. As a result, the meat, fish, and seafood proportion of the human diet rose.

Around this time, an important genetic mutation occurred. Some humans acquired the ability to digest lactose. They could drink milk and eat dairy foods after weaning. Three out of four Americans are estimated to be able to digest lactose, but only one in four people worldwide can. Today many Americans consume a majority of their calories from animal foods and grains, something that would have been impossible just five hundred generations ago.

During the nineteenth and twentieth centuries, anthropologists documented the lives of the few remaining hunter-gatherer groups. They had no modern antibiotics and typically died young of infectious diseases. But some lived into old age. Hunter-gatherer elders were remarkably free of the chronic health problems that plague us today: heart disease, cancer, obesity, diabetes, high blood pressure—and osteoporosis.

In Dr. Cordain's words, "we are genetic Stone Agers living in the Space Age." As a species, we're genetically programmed to thrive on a diet of fruits, vegetables, seeds, and nuts. These foods are alkaline and contribute to strong bones—and prevention of heart disease, cancer, and other contemporary health problems. In evolutionary terms, animal foods and grains are dietary newcomers. They provide calories and many nutrients. But they also come with drawbacks—saturated fat (meats) and acid blood (meats and grains). As a result, foods central to the diets of North Americans, Europeans, and a growing proportion of the rest of the world cause osteoporosis. Human evolution has not caught up with what agriculture and a chance mutation have done to the human diet.

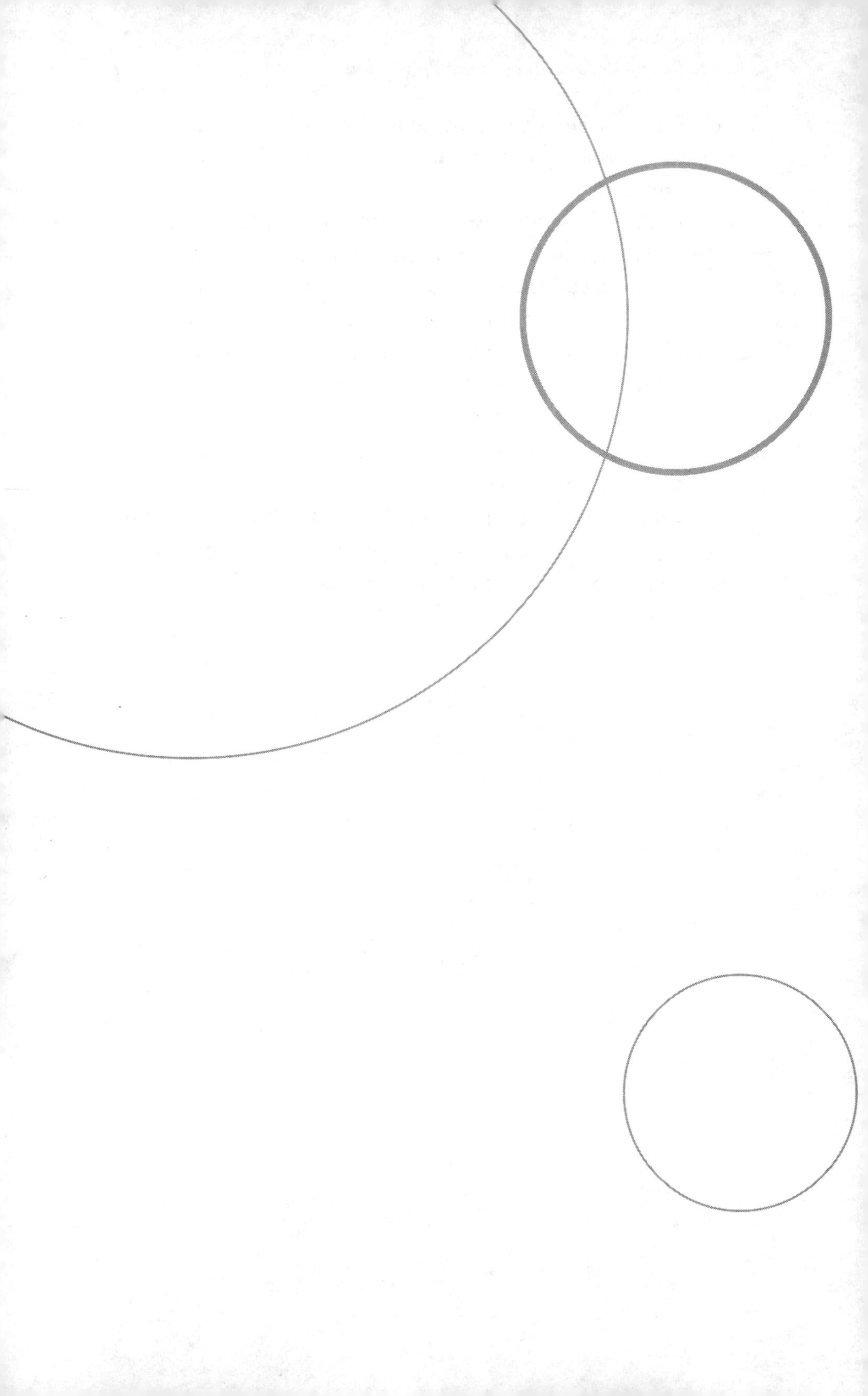

Why a Forty-Year-Old Explanation Is "New"

One of us (MC) is married to a doctor, many of whose patients have osteoporosis. Like all physicians, she must attend continuing medical education seminars. During the writing of this book she attended two. Both featured updates on osteoporosis.

At one a distinguished professor at a prestigious medical school recommended milk, dairy, calcium, exercise, and drugs. At the other another eminent professor from another well-known medical school recommended milk, dairy, calcium, *not too much protein*, and drugs. One said nothing about low-acid eating. The other mentioned it in passing.

The bad news is that many osteoporosis experts are apparently unaware of or unmoved by the mountain of evidence refuting the calcium theory. The good news is that the low-acid theory is finally emerging from the rarefied confines of research laboratories into the practice of medicine.

This change is happening much too slowly. With so much evidence against milk, dairy, and calcium, why do so many experts still cling to a bankrupt theory? And with so much evidence in favor of low-acid eating, why isn't it more widely accepted? We're not sure. But we have some ideas.

How Paradigms Shift

The myth is that science marches resolutely forward, that researchers quickly incorporate new findings into accepted scientific theories (paradigms). This is often not the case.

A scientific paradigm is like the brick house in "The Three Little Pigs." Once a paradigm becomes established, it's hard to blow down. Of course, no paradigm answers every question. Over time evidence that contradicts the accepted theory may accumulate. Yet the paradigm continues to be invoked as the accepted explanation. Then at some point, a tipping point, a metaphorical earthquake strikes, shattering the paradigm's house into a pile of rubble, and a new paradigm replaces it.

This process can take centuries. Five hundred years before Columbus, Arab philosophers insisted that the Earth was round. But the Catholic Church clung to the view that the planet was flat. When Columbus sailed west from Spain, he was confident he would not fall off the end of the Earth. But some of his crew feared otherwise. It took until 1522 to prove once and for all that the Earth is round. That was the year a remnant of Ferdinand Magellan's crew returned to Spain after successfully circumnavigating the globe.

In the modern world, paradigms shift more quickly, but they still take time, often decades. Cigarette smoking became fashionable in the United States around World War I. By World War II studies showed that, compared with nonsmokers, longtime smokers had a much higher risk of lung cancer. But the paradigm did not shift decisively until twenty years later, in 1964, when the surgeon general first declared that smoking causes lung cancer. And it took another generation for smoking to be banned in most public places.

For the past twenty years, we've been witnessing a slow paradigm shift on global warming. In the 1980s, when the idea was first advanced, many scientists scoffed. Some still do. But a new paradigm has basically been established, one that seeks to limit greenhouse gases and carbon footprints. (Low-acid eating helps; see Chapter 17.)

The low-acid paradigm was first articulated in 1968. Over the past forty years evidence has slowly accumulated that the calcium theory is invalid, that the low-acid paradigm offers a more compelling explanation of osteoporosis.

The low-acid paradigm is a long way from acceptance. It's about where global warming was around, say, 1990. But slowly it's becoming more accepted.

The Primacy of Protein

Low-acid eating means cutting back substantially on meat, fish, poultry, and cheese. This is a key reason for its remaining in the wilderness. To many Americans—and residents of other countries with epidemic levels of osteoporosis—eating less of these foods is almost inconceivable, like swimming without water. A substantial proportion of the population assumes that a high-protein diet is a boon to health. Animal foods are high in protein. Therefore, animal foods must be good.

Protein, carbohydrates, and fat were first identified as the three components of food by the English chemist William Prout (1785–1850). He was mistaken. He knew nothing of vitamins and minerals, antioxidants and fiber. The German scientist Justus von Liebig (1803–1873), often called the father of nutrition science, added minerals to Prout's list and declared the mystery of nutrition solved. He, too, was mistaken, missing vitamins, antioxidants, and fiber. But von Liebig did not allow ignorance to prevent pontification. He proclaimed protein the "master nutrient" because he believed (mistakenly) that it alone controlled growth.

Nutrition writer Michael Pollan notes: "To a considerable extent, we still have a food system organized around the promotion of protein as the master nutrient." As a result, meat and dairy foods are generally assumed to be good for health, despite overwhelming scientific evidence that a diet based on them substantially increases risk of many of the conditions that plague today's Americans: obesity, high blood pressure, heart disease, stroke, cancer, diabetes, Alzheimer's disease—and osteoporosis.

In actuality, humans need only a small portion of calories daily to come from protein—about 10 percent. For a person who needs about 2,000 calories per day to meet his or her energy needs, that is only 50 grams of protein a day, less than two ounces, about half of a chicken breast. An even more precise way to determine your protein need is to multiply your body weight by 0.36 g/lb weight (or 0.8 g/kg weight). For a 140-pound person that would be 0.36 grams per pound multiplied by 140 pounds, 50.9 grams. Most Americans currently consume protein in quantities well beyond their needs.

The Culture of Affluence

Most Americans and many people around the world can't conceive of eating less meat and dairy for another reason, the belief that affluence *entitles* them to a diet overflowing with these foods. Meat, poultry, fish, seafood, cheese, and ice cream are viewed as perks of the good life.

Our evolutionary ancestors were hunter-gatherers, but they did much more gathering than hunting. Have you ever tried to hunt? It's very difficult, even with telescopic sights on modern weapons. It was nearly impossible for our prehuman ancestors, who had no weapons. It wasn't much easier for early humans, who had stone-tipped spears and arrows. As a result, our ancestors ate meat only occasionally. They also lacked refrigeration, so what little meat they hunted or scavenged quickly rotted.

As agriculture developed, meat, milk, and egg consumption increased (except among most Asians and many Africans, many of whom lack the mutation that allows digestion of lactose). But the vast majority of people still ate a plant-based diet, consuming meat only on special occasions.

Until the twentieth century the large majority of Americans lived on small farms. If they were well off, they had a cow or two for milk, a few pigs for meat, and some chickens for eggs and occasionally meat. But they did not eat meat daily. They couldn't afford to. For most people, meat was reserved for special occasions, notably Sunday dinner, when a chicken or some ham or bacon might be served alongside the family's standard fare: potatoes, beans, greens, vegetable soups and stews, and bread or corn bread, with fruit for dessert (fresh or home-canned), or perhaps a fruit pie.

In the twentieth century meat production became industrialized, and refrigeration and freezing allowed extended food storage and long-distance shipping. As a result, meat production rose and prices fell. As Americans became more affluent, they ate more of it, especially after World War II. According to the U.S. Department of Agriculture (USDA), in 1950 annual per-capita consumption of chicken, turkey, veal, lamb, beef, and pork came to 144 pounds. By 2007, despite a mountain of research linking meat consumption to chronic diseases, the figure had increased 54 percent to 220 pounds.

Dairy consumption has also increased. Milk drinking has declined (largely replaced by soft drinks), but cheese consumption has tripled—from eleven pounds per American per year to thirty-one pounds in just over thirty years.

Today the same thing is happening around the world. As formerly impoverished nations become more affluent, their populations can afford more meat and cheese—and buy them enthusiastically. They feel entitled. In 1990, McDonald's had three thousand restaurants outside the United States. Today the company boasts more than fifteen thousand in 117 countries, and four out of five new McDonald's are opened outside the United States. Once the world's most widely recognized commercial brand was Coca-Cola. Today it's the golden arches.

"When people become better off," writes Marion Nestle, Ph.D., the Paulette Goddard professor of nutrition, food studies, and public health at New York University, in her book *Food Politics*, "they abandon traditional plant-based diets and eat more meat, fat, and processed foods. The result is a sharp increase in chronic diseases."

"If you're poor," notes T. Colin Campbell, the Jacob Gould Schulman professor of nutritional biochemistry at Cornell University and author of *The China Study*, "you eat plant foods. If you're rich, you eat meat."

How One USDA Mission Trumps Another—to the Detriment of Health

For almost a century, the U.S. government has encouraged Americans to eat animal foods. In 1862, Congress created the USDA and gave it two missions—to assure a reliable food supply by supporting U.S. agriculture and to "diffuse among the people useful information on subjects connected with agriculture in the most general sense of the word." As a result, the USDA became a primary provider of diet and nutrition advice.

The USDA's twin missions have caused conflict. The agency encouraged tobacco farming long after it had been linked indisputably to lung cancer. The USDA no longer promotes tobacco. But it actively supports dairy farming and cattle ranching and continues to trumpet milk, dairy foods, and meat as essential to a healthful diet, despite the enormous amount of medical evidence to the contrary.

In 1917, the USDA issued its first dietary recommendations, urging Americans to select foods from five groups: (1) vegetables, which included fruits; (2) cereals, breads, and grains; (3) milk and meats; (4) sugary foods; and (5) fatty foods.

Food groups have been with us ever since. There was no science behind the creations of these groups. They were simply a convenient way to discuss food—while bolstering the USDA's primary mission, promotion of American agriculture, no matter what American farmers grew.

In 1942, to strengthen the nation for World War II, the USDA recommended seven food groups: (1) milk and dairy products; (2) meats, poultry, fish, eggs, beans, and peas; (3) tomatoes and citrus fruits; (4) green and yellow vegetables; (5) potatoes and other vegetables and fruits; (6) flours, cereals, and breads; and (7) butter and margarine.

In 1956, the USDA released its best-known guidelines, the Basic Four Food Groups: (1) milk and dairy products, (2) meats, (3) fruits and vegetables, and (4) grains.

With every revision, the USDA based its recommendations not on science but on promoting consumption of U.S. agricultural products.

By the 1970s it was clear that red meat and whole-milk dairy foods were key contributors to heart disease and many cancers. Health officials demanded more science-based diet recommendations. In 1977, the Senate Select Committee on Nutrition and Human Needs held hearings and produced a seminal report, *Dietary Goals for the United States*. It advised eating more fruits and vegetables and less meat, milk, and dairy foods.

Dairy farmers and cattle ranchers were outraged. Political pressure forced the Senate Select Committee to back away from recommending less meat, milk, and dairy. Since then, no U.S. government publication has ever encouraged Americans to limit meat and dairy foods.

Meanwhile, nutrition advocates continued to demand science-based food guidelines. In 1986, the U.S. surgeon general convened a group of experts to craft them. Marion Nestle was one of them. "My first day on the job, I was given the rules. No matter what the research indicated, the report could not recommend 'eat less meat.' "

The meat and dairy industries have great influence with the USDA. But they don't own it. Nutrition activists and fruit and vegetable growers also influence the agency. In 1989, the USDA reorganized its food groups once again, this time incorporating some science. It expanded the list from four groups to five, reintroducing fats and sweets. It also organized the groups into a pyramid to suggest how much of each group should be consumed. The pyramid did not discourage meat and dairy. But it suggested more daily servings of fruits, vegetables, grains, and breads. (See Figure 8.1.)

The meat and dairy industries were outraged. It didn't matter that the pyramid recommended two to three daily servings of milk, yogurt, cheese, meat, poultry, and fish. By recommending more fruits and vegetables than animal foods, animal food producers considered it a disaster.

Meat and dairy advocates wanted the pyramid changed. That happened in 2005. (See Figure 8.2 on page 93.) The current pyramid is considerably less informative. Without reading the fine print, it's difficult to know how much of each group to eat.

FIGURE 8.1 Food Guide Pyramid: A Guide to Daily Food Choices

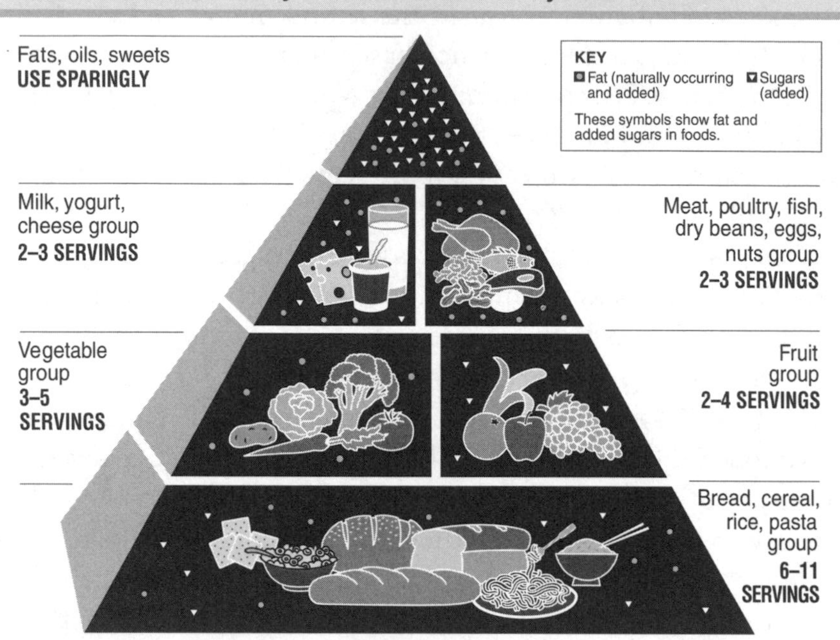

Source: U.S. Department of Agriculture/U.S. Department of Health and Human Services, August 1992

Only one agency has found a way to buck the meat and dairy lobbies. In 1991, the National Cancer Institute launched its "5 A Day" program. The NCI asks everyone to eat at least five daily servings of fruits and vegetables, preferably six to nine. The NCI doesn't mention meat or dairy, so the agency triggered no controversy over calls to eat less of them. All the NCI recommended was a minimum of five daily servings of fruits and vegetables. This is a good start for low-acid eating. Unfortunately, the NCI has spent at most only $3 million a year to promote its 5 A Day program—just 1 cent per person in the United States. Compared with the marketing muscle (to the tune of $150 million per year) behind "Got Milk?" that's nothing.

Publication and Publicity Bias

The final reason why the low-acid theory remains under the radar is that many studies supporting it show that something *does not*

FIGURE 8.2 MyPyramid: Steps to a Healthier You

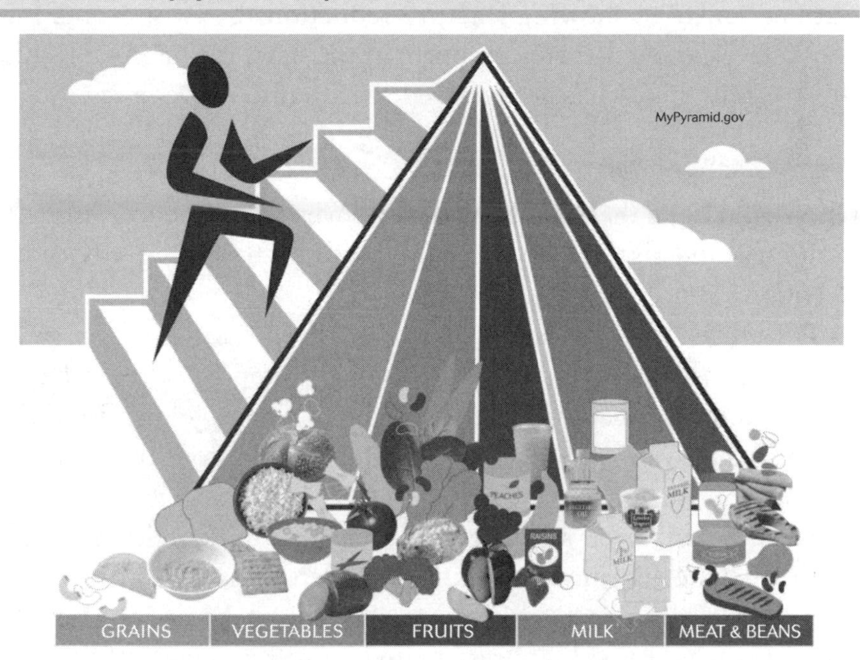

happen: no decrease in fracture risk with milk, dairy, and calcium. Studies are much more likely to get published—and publicized—when they show that something happens. When nothing happens, that's of less interest to medical journal editors and the news media. Researchers call this publication and publicity bias.

As you now know, since 1975, forty-seven studies have shown that milk, dairy, and calcium reduce fracture risk. That's more than one per year. Many have been widely publicized, which helps explain why the conventional wisdom is still generally regarded as true.

As you know as well, since 1975, ninety-four studies have refuted the conventional wisdom. These studies have garnered much less publicity. Only one has made headlines, the prospective trial involving 36,282 postmenopausal women followed for seven years that showed no benefit from calcium and/or vitamin D. (See Chapter 5.)

Studies showing no benefit for milk, dairy, and calcium vastly outnumber those showing fracture reductions by two to one. But you'd never know that from reports in the news media. As a result, the low-acid theory has not received the attention it deserves.

We're Disappointed

One would hope that health authorities who make diet recommendations would rise above cultural biases and base their advice on nutrition science. Alas, they have not.

Fortunately, the situation is changing. The low-acid theory is gaining momentum. The research increasingly supports a plant-based diet for bone health. Many scientists who not long ago dismissed the low-acid theory have changed their minds. And at continuing medical education seminars, doctors just might hear about it.

Nonetheless, given all the evidence against milk, dairy, and calcium, and the enormous amount of evidence in favor of low-acid eating, we're disappointed in those who advise Americans how to prevent osteoporosis. It appears many are still prisoners of the cultural bias in favor of a high-protein animal food-based diet. They have not kept up with the medical literature.

Bricks and Mortar: For Strong Bones, the Body Needs More than Calcium

IMAGINE TWO BRICK walls. One contains a hundred bricks but very little mortar. The other contains only sixty bricks but lots of mortar. The wall with a hundred bricks is larger. But is it stronger?

Imagine that cars hit both walls at the same speed. One wall shatters. The other holds. Which wall crumbled?

The one without much mortar. Why? Because the strength of a brick wall depends not only on its brick, but also on how well they're cemented. A brick wall without much mortar is little more than a pile of loose bricks.

If Calcium Improves BMD, Why Doesn't It Prevent Fractures?

So far you've read about three of the four types of studies that have been done to investigate the cause(s) of osteoporosis: prospective trials, retrospective trials, and meta-analyses. This chapter focuses on the bone mineral density (BMD) research, studies of the mineral content of bone, which presumably is crucial to its strength. In BMD studies, researchers measure BMD over time, following subjects' diet and lifestyle and correlating any differences, or measure subjects' BMD and then ask participants to make a change, like taking calcium pills, and then retest subjects' BMD to see if the intervention has made any difference.

As already mentioned, BMD studies are cheaper, easier, and quicker than prospective and retrospective trials correlating milk, dairy, and calcium intake with fractures. Therefore many more of them—214 compared to 140 since 1975—have been published. This is what they've shown:

- One hundred eleven studies (52 percent) show that milk, dairy, and calcium increase BMD.
- Forty-one trials (19 percent) are inconclusive.
- Sixty-two studies (29 percent) show that milk, dairy, and calcium have no effect on BMD.

The calcium theory wins by a score of 52 to 48 percent. This is a victory for the conventional wisdom. But just barely.

It's not particularly compelling—here's why:

- Milk, dairy, and calcium increase BMD *only* in premenopausal women. In postmenopausal women, they simply slow bone loss. Instead of suffering a hip fracture at seventy-eight, milk, dairy, and calcium might postpone it until age eighty-two. That's good, but it's no cure.
- As we've seen, no matter what milk, dairy, and calcium do for BMD, they don't prevent the outcome that matters most to the public health. *They don't prevent fractures.* This is the biggest concern with these studies.

Common sense says that if BMD improves, bones should become stronger and less likely to fracture. Apparently not. Why doesn't improved BMD prevent fractures?

Bone Mineral Density Reconsidered

Let's go back to the two brick walls. If you think of the bricks as calcium and the mortar as all the other nutrients crucial to building strong bones, the wall with a hundred bricks corresponds to bones in the West. Americans, Canadians, Western Europeans, Australians, and New Zealanders have high calcium consumption and high BMD—lots of bricks. But they have the world's highest fracture rates. They must be short on mortar.

The wall with sixty bricks corresponds to bones in much of the rest of the world. Other countries have lower BMD—fewer bricks—but fracture rates much lower than ours. They must have lots of mortar.

Our health authorities insist that by gorging on calcium, we gain stronger bones. In fact, all we do is pile a few more loose bricks on the wall—without much mortar. The wall becomes slightly larger—*but no stronger.* In fact, it's weaker than the smaller wall whose bricks are well cemented.

To build strong bones, we need more than just bricks. We also need mortar—and lots of it.

Beyond Calcium: It Takes Seventeen Other Nutrients to Build Strong Bones

If bones were just sticks of calcium, they would be chalk. But they're not. Bones are living cells (mature osteoblasts) held immobile in a lattice of protein-rich collagen whose spongelike spaces are filled by crystals of hardened calcium compounds and other minerals.

If BMD measured only calcium, it would be called bone *calcium* density. However, this test measures not just calcium, but *all* the minerals in bone, and does not distinguish between bricks and mortar. These other minerals include:

- **Boron.** Without enough, the body cannot efficiently use calcium, magnesium, and vitamin D to make strong bones.

- **Copper.** Necessary for collagen formation and bone mineralization. Low levels increase risk of osteoporosis.

- **Fluoride.** Helps harden the minerals in bones and teeth.

- **Magnesium.** Without it, vitamin D can't move calcium into bone. Magnesium deficiency is a major risk factor for osteoporosis.

- **Manganese.** Necessary for both collagen formation and bone mineralization. Deficiency is a major risk factor for fractures.

- **Phosphorus.** For strong bones, calcium must combine with phosphorus.

- **Silica (Silicon).** Necessary for crystallization of calcium.

- **Zinc.** Helps build the collagen framework for bone.

In addition to minerals, strong bones require many vitamins:

- **Vitamin A.** Bone-building osteoblasts cannot develop properly without it.

- **Vitamin C.** Necessary for the formation of bone collagen.

- **Vitamin B_6.** Without enough, bones are weak.

- **Vitamin B_{12}.** Osteoblasts cannot build bone without it.

- **Vitamin D.** By itself or with calcium, it's no osteoporosis cure. It is necessary, but not sufficient, to build bone strength. Vitamin D is needed for incorporation of calcium and phosphorus into bone, and many studies show that people who suffer osteoporotic fractures have low levels.

- **Vitamin K.** Crucial to incorporation of mineral crystals into the collagen matrix. Low levels increase fracture risk.

- **Folic acid.** Helps prevent bone demineralization.

Finally, strong bones require:

- **Essential fatty acids.** These good fats are necessary for a healthy collagen matrix and for normal bone mineralization.

- **Protein.** Although a flood of poorly buffered amino acids from animal protein destroys bone, a modest amount of protein is a key component of bone's collagen matrix.

These seventeen nutrients are not only necessary for strong bones but also must also be consumed *in the proper proportions.* For example, without enough vitamin A, bones cannot develop normally. But too much *increases* fracture risk, as discussed later in this chapter.

Before you check the label on your vitamins to make sure they contain all these nutrients, know that you don't need supplements to obtain them. With the exception of vitamin B_{12}, all these nutrients can be found easily, affordably, and in the proper proportions in the foods humans evolved to thrive on—fruits, vegetables, nuts, and legumes.

Beyond Alkaline Buffering: Fruits and Vegetables Also Supply Essential Bone-Building Nutrients

Recall that fruits and vegetables are alkaline. Eat lots of them and the body has no need to draw calcium from bone to buffer the acids formed by meats, milk, dairy foods, and grains. But there's another reason to eat a diet based on fruits and vegetables. Unlike high-protein foods, they contain all the other nutrients essential for strong bones, except vitamin B_{12}.

Compared with animal foods, fruits and vegetables are much richer in the "mortar" nutrients necessary for strong bones. The evidence is in the BMD studies. Compared with milk, dairy, and calcium, fruits and vegetables improve BMD *much more effectively.*

Researchers have published 103 studies on the BMD effects of fruits and vegetables—or on the effects of nutrients found only or primarily in them, such as antioxidants. The first appeared in 1988. A dozen were published in the 1990s as the low-acid theory began to attract research interest. But the vast majority have appeared since 2000, as the low-acid theory has gained momentum. These studies have attracted little media attention, but their results are impressive:

- Eighty-seven of the 103 studies (84 percent) show that as fruit and vegetable or antioxidant consumption increases, so does BMD.
- Nine trials (9 percent) are inconclusive.
- Seven (7 percent) show that fruits and vegetables have no effect on BMD.

While only a slim majority of studies, just 52 percent, show that milk, dairy, and calcium improve bone mineral density, the vast majority of studies, a whopping 84 percent, show that fruits and vegetables boost BMD. *The most reliable way to improve bone mineral density is to eat more fruits and vegetables.*

The Best Fruit, Vegetable, Nut, and Legume Sources of "Mortar" Nutrients

Here are good fruit-and-vegetable sources of mortar nutrients:

- **Boron.** All fruits and vegetables contain some.
- **Copper.** Beans, raisins, and nuts
- **Fluoride.** Tea, beans, potatoes, and carrots
- **Magnesium.** Potatoes, soy foods, seeds, nuts, beans, bananas, oranges, tomatoes, spinach, lettuce, chard, and kale
- **Manganese.** Avocados, seeds, and nuts, especially pecans and hazelnuts
- **Phosphorus.** Beans and nuts
- **Silica (Silicon).** Coffee and all fruits and vegetables

- **Zinc.** Beans, especially peanuts

- **Vitamin A.** Carrots, cantaloupe, apricots, spinach, sweet potatoes, yams, kale, and greens

- **Vitamin B_6.** Carrots, spinach, peas, walnuts, sunflower seeds, cabbage, cantaloupe, avocados, bananas, and beans

- **Vitamin C.** Oranges, lemons, limes, bananas, cantaloupe, strawberries, bell peppers, broccoli, asparagus, cauliflower, potatoes, and tomatoes

- **Vitamin D.** Mushrooms, as discussed later in this chapter. But the main source is the body's production in the skin in response to sunlight.

- **Vitamin K.** The richest sources are lettuce, spinach, chard, cabbage, broccoli, and collard and turnip greens.

- **Folic acid.** Spinach, broccoli, asparagus, chard, kale, and beet greens.

- **Essential fatty acids.** Walnuts and pumpkin seeds

- **Protein.** All fruits and vegetables contain some. The richest plant sources are beans, nuts, seeds, and soy foods.

There's no need to obsess about eating these specific fruits and vegetables. Just eat a wide variety of fruits and vegetables. Have fruits and vegetables at every meal. Eat a serving of beans or peas daily and snack on fruit and nuts.

The one mortar nutrient that cannot be found in plant foods is vitamin B_{12} (cobalamin). Vegans can obtain it from supplements and fortified cereals. Ovo-lacto-vegetarians can get it from milk, cheese, and eggs. Salmon and sardines also contain B_{12}. Omnivores can obtain it from beef and organ meats (liver, kidney). You don't need much. One or two servings of animal foods per month is sufficient.

Supplement or Produce Aisle: Where Should You Shop?

When Americans see lists of nutrients, they often head not to the produce section but to the supplement aisle. The mortar nutrients can, indeed, be obtained from supplements—and vegans may have to get their vitamin B_{12} that way. But for strong bones and lower risk of fractures, heart disease, cancer, Alzheimer's, and other chronic conditions, it's best to obtain these nutrients from fruits, vegetables, and other products.

We have nothing against one-a-day vitamins as a form of nutritional health insurance—just in case you don't get enough of something from food. For example, selenium is an antioxidant that reduces the risk of several cancers. But soils differ greatly in selenium content. So do the foods grown in them. Few of us know the selenium content of our fruits and vegetables, so it's prudent to take a one-a-day supplement that contains it. But vitamins *do not* make up for eating fewer than five daily servings of fruits and vegetables—and preferably six to nine.

It's best to get your calcium and mortar nutrients not from pills but from fruits and vegetables—for many reasons:

- **Even if you take every supplement available, you get only a tiny fraction of necessary nutrients.** Consider vitamin A. It's not a single nutrient, but a huge family of them, the carotenoids, including more than 600 compounds. The vast majority of supplements contain only one carotenoid, beta-carotene. But all 600 are important to good health. Perhaps you've heard of lycopene, found in tomatoes. It reduces risk of prostate cancer. Lycopene is a carotenoid available in supplements. If you take a multivitamin with beta-carotene and lycopene, you get two of the 600 carotenoids. How can you obtain the other 598? Eat a wide variety of green and yellow-orange fruits and vegetables, including carrots, yams, sweet potatoes, cantaloupe, apricots, parsley, spinach, and kale.

- **Supplements are isolated nutrients.** They do not supply much of the alkaline material necessary for strong bones. Fruits and vegetables are bulkier. They contain the alkaline material that maintains optimal blood pH.

- **Fruits and vegetables contain nutrients in the proportions best for good health.** Humans evolved to function best on the combinations of nutrients found naturally in fruits and vegetables. Too much of one supplemental nutrient can interfere with the metabolism of others. The easiest, cheapest, safest way to get enough of all of them in the proper proportions is to eat lots of fruits and vegetables.

- **It's very difficult to ingest bone-harming high levels of vitamin A from food.** It's easy to overdose on vitamin A from supplements; see the discussion later in this chapter.

- **Finally, a great deal of research shows that a diet high in fruits and vegetables substantially reduces the risk of not just osteoporosis but also death from all causes.** Some studies show similar benefits from certain supplements. But the supplement research is nowhere near as consistent as the enormous literature on diets high in fruits and vegetables. Take a supplement if you like. But for a long, healthy life with a low risk of osteoporosis, heart disease, cancer, diabetes, Alzheimer's disease, and other conditions, eat at least five servings of fruits and vegetables a day—and the more the better.

The Osteoporosis Cure

"Fruits and Vegetables: The Unexpected Natural Answer to Osteoporosis Prevention?" That's the title of an editorial in the *American Journal of Clinical Nutrition* by Susan A. New, Ph.D., a researcher at the Center for Nutrition and Food Safety at the University of Surrey in England. She writes: "We urgently need public health strategies to maintain bone health throughout life and to prevent osteoporosis in later life. The evidence from many studies strongly points to a positive link between fruit and vegetable consumption and bone health. A fruit-and-vegetables approach provides a very sensible and natural approach to osteoporosis prevention, one that is likely to have numerous additional benefits [less obesity, diabetes, high blood pressure, heart disease, cancer, and Alzheimer's]. However, persuading Western populations to increase their fruit and vegetable consumption remains our biggest challenge."

Vitamin D: What You Need to Know About This Crucial Bone Builder

Until recently, scientists believed vitamin D was not available from plant foods. However, in the past few years, mushrooms have been shown to contain substantial amounts. To date, only a few studies have been published. As this book goes to press, it's still not clear whether mushrooms can supply enough vitamin D for strong bones. Fortunately, there are other ways to obtain it.

Vitamin D is the one bone-building nutrient we make ourselves. When exposed to ultraviolet sunlight, special cells in the skin make this vitamin. To make healthy amounts, it takes fifteen to twenty minutes of sun on the face, neck, and arms three times a week with the sun at least forty-five degrees above the horizon—you have to look up, but not much.

Sunscreens interfere with vitamin D synthesis because they prevent ultraviolet light from hitting the skin. If you use sunscreen during a day at the beach, consider not using it if you go outdoors only briefly. Note: Many cosmetics contain sunscreen, so women who use them should consider this when budgeting time in the sun.

After age fifty, the body's ability to make vitamin D declines. As a result, deficiency is common in the elderly, especially among those with fractures.

In northern latitudes, during winter, it's difficult for the skin to make vitamin D. Several studies in New England, England, and Scandinavia have documented seasonal variations, with levels dipping into the deficiency zone in winter. In the United States, the line of demarcation is 40° north latitude. North of this line—roughly from Philadelphia through Columbus, Ohio, Topeka, and Denver, to Sacramento—vitamin D deficiency is a problem in winter. As a result, it's often prudent to supplement this nutrient. The standard recommendation is 400 to 800 IU a day.

But be careful. Intake greater than 2,000 IU a day may cause problems. Signs of too much include fatigue, nausea, headache, restlessness, diarrhea, and loss of appetite.

Body levels of vitamin D can be determined with a blood test. If you're concerned about yours, ask your physician for the test.

Vitamin K: The Rodney Dangerfield of Nutrients

All fruits and vegetables help build bone, but lettuce, spinach, dark leafy greens (chard, collard greens, turnip greens, etc.), green cabbage, and broccoli are particularly valuable because they are rich in vitamin K.

Vitamin K gets no respect. It's not included in many one-a-day vitamin/mineral formulas. But it has major impact on bone health. Many studies show that low levels of vitamin K are associated with low BMD. In addition, six of seven fracture trials (86 percent) show that this vitamin reduces fracture risk, often substantially. A few examples:

- Harvard researchers surveyed dietary intake of vitamin K in 72,327 nurses and then followed them for ten years. Compared with those who ate no more than one serving of lettuce a week, those who ate lettuce daily were 45 percent less likely to suffer a hip fracture.
- Tufts researchers tracked the diets and fractures of 888 participants in the Framingham Heart Study for seven years. Compared with those who consumed the least vitamin K, those who ate the most had 65 percent less risk of hip fracture.
- British researchers conducted a meta-analysis of studies of vitamin K for fracture prevention. Compared with participants who had the lowest blood levels of the vitamin, those who had the highest levels enjoyed a whopping 77 percent lower risk of hip fracture.

Too Much Vitamin A *Increases* Fracture Risk

Five of seven studies (71 percent) show that high blood levels of vitamin A reduce BMD and increase risk of fractures.

Among the studies showing increased fracture risk, three are prospective trials. They average 29,545 participants followed for an average of twenty-three years—big numbers for a very long time.

Both studies showing no increased fracture risk from vitamin A are also prospective, averaging 18,655 participants followed for an average of 6.6 years—fewer trials with smaller numbers for considerably less time, so less persuasive.

The weight of the evidence shows that excessive consumption of vitamin A decreases BMD and boosts fracture risk.

But what exactly is "excessive" intake? Enough to turn white and Asian skin noticeably orange, a condition called *carotenemia*. In people with very dark skin, the skin of the palms and soles of the feet turn orange. If you develop carotenemia, stop taking vitamin A supplements unless a physician prescribes them. It would also be prudent to cut down on carrots, cantaloupe, apricots, spinach, sweet potatoes, yams, kale, and greens.

However, for most Americans, even those who take vitamin A pills, carotenemia is not an issue. The typical American consumes *too few* fruits and vegetables containing vitamin A.

Soy Foods Increase Bone Mineral Density

Table 7.1 (on page 58) shows that beans have unpredictable effects on blood and urine acidity. Some are acid producing, while others are alkaline. But a good deal of research shows that soy foods, including tofu, are alkaline bone builders.

Thirty-one clinical trials have been published on the effects of soy foods on BMD:

- Twenty-two (71 percent) show that they increase BMD. A prospective study of 24,403 postmenopausal women followed for 4.5 years shows that a high-soy diet also reduces risk of fractures.
- Five studies (16 percent) are inconclusive.
- Four (13 percent) show no bone-building effect for soy.

The weight of the evidence—almost three-quarters of trials—shows that soy foods improve BMD. This is important because soy foods can be used as tasty substitutes for meat in many dishes. (See Chapter 11.)

Bone Mineral Density: A Second-Rate Test

There's just no getting around the fact that BMD testing has a major shortcoming. When it increases, fracture risk does not necessarily fall. Osteoporosis researchers have known this for quite a while. In a recent review of BMD testing, R. E. Small of Virginia Commonwealth University in Richmond concludes: "There is a poor correlation between BMD increases and fracture risk reduction." And in an essay in the *Journal of the American Medical Association*, University of Toronto researchers A. M. Cheung and A. S. Detsky note: "BMD is only one determinant of bone strength. Many [other] factors that contribute to bone strength are not captured by BMD. Recent data suggest that falls are a stronger predictor of fractures than BMD."

Falls are a better predictor because more than 95 percent of hip fractures in the elderly and many wrist, arm, and other fractures are triggered by falls. (See Chapter 13.)

Osteoporosis was once diagnosed when a fracture occurred. A predictive test was sorely needed to see who was at risk. In the 1980s, a special x-ray was developed to measure bone mineral density. In 1993, the UN's World Health Organization (WHO) enshrined it as the gold standard by declaring that osteoporosis should be diagnosed if BMD fell below certain statistical criteria.

Suddenly doctors began ordering BMD tests for women as young as forty—and prescribing drugs for those with readings even modestly below normal. But even in the heyday of BMD testing, some authorities remained skeptical. The U.S. Preventive Services

continued

Task Force, an expert panel convened by the Department of Health and Human Services, recommends routine BMD testing *only* for women aged sixty-five and older, or beginning at age sixty for women who are at high risk for fractures because of family history or early menopause.

Recently WHO expanded its diagnostic criteria beyond low BMD with a new standard Fracture Risk Assessment, also known as FRAX, that estimates the likelihood of suffering a fracture over the next ten years. The FRAX standard uses BMD, but it includes other risk factors as well, including age, gender, height, weight, personal and family history of fractures, smoking, and alcohol consumption.

As this book goes to press, the FRAX test is just beginning to be adopted by physicians. Future studies will determine whether it's a significant improvement over BMD testing—whether it works in both directions. We hope it does. Second-rate BMD testing should be replaced with a first-rate test, one that reliably predicts fracture risk. Preventing fractures is what counts. That's why throughout this book we have focused on fractures and not on BMD, except in this chapter.

When it comes to boosting BMD, barely half the studies show that milk, dairy, and calcium are effective. Meanwhile, a far more convincing 84 percent of trials show that fruits and vegetables enhance BMD. With fruits and vegetables improving bone mineral density so much better than milk, dairy, and calcium, you might think we would be touting BMD testing as compelling evidence in favor of low-acid eating.

But the fact is, BMD is a second-rate test. It's not a very good indicator of bone health because it works well only in one direction.

An example of a first-rate medical test is blood pressure. As blood pressure rises, heart attack and stroke become more likely. As blood pressure declines, these risks subside. Blood pressure testing provides meaningful, real-world results in both directions, as readings rise or fall.

There is no doubt that when BMD falls below a certain point, fractures become more likely. But BMD testing does not work very well in the opposite direction. As BMD rises, risk of fracture *does not reliably decline.*

Consider:

- Milk, dairy foods, and calcium supplements increase BMD significantly in 52 percent of studies. However, they reduce fracture risk in only 33 percent of studies.
- Asians have lower BMD than whites. But Asians also have lower rates of osteoporotic fractures.
- Drinking tea increases BMD. But some trials show that tea (and other beverages containing caffeine) have either no effect on fracture risk or increase it. (See Chapter 15.)
- The drugs used to treat osteoporosis all increase BMD. But some of them do not reduce risk of various fractures (Chapter 16).

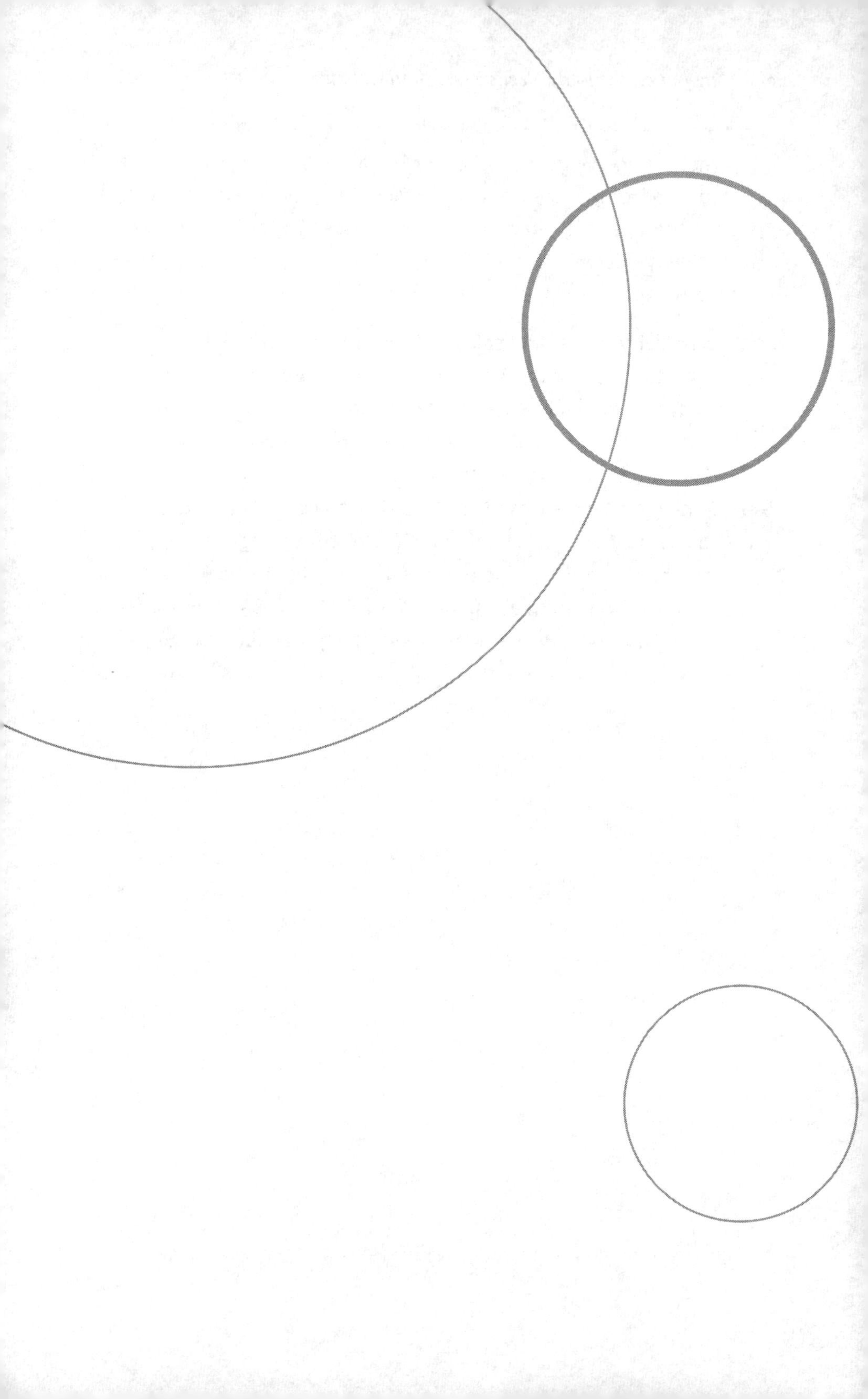

The Case Against Low-Acid Eating

If critics wanted to refute low-acid eating, their prayers would be answered by studies that showed either that a diet high in animal protein *reduces* fracture risk or that a vegan diet *increases* it. As it happens, four such studies have been published: three reporting reduced risk of fractures with increasing meat consumption and one showing that vegans suffer more fractures than meat eaters:

- Utah State researchers surveyed the diets of 41,837 postmenopausal Iowa women and then surveyed them again three years later. Those who ate the most protein suffered the fewest fractures. "Animal protein appeared to account for the difference."
- Another group of Utah State scientists identified 1,167 Utah residents over fifty who'd suffered hip fractures and compared their diets with those of 1,334 matched controls who had not. As total protein consumption increased, risk of hip fracture decreased significantly.
- At Loma Linda University in southern California, researchers surveyed the diets of 1,685 women over forty and then surveyed them again twenty-five years later, correlating their diets and

wrist fractures. "Increasing meat consumption decreased the risk of wrist fracture."

- Oxford University researchers surveyed the diets of 34,696 adults and then followed them for five years. Meat eaters, fish eaters, and ovo-lacto-vegetarians had virtually the same fracture rate, but vegans suffered 15 percent more fractures.

On closer examination, two of these trials are open to question:

- In the study involving Utah residents, a diet high in animal protein reduced fractures *only* in those aged fifty to sixty-nine. For participants aged seventy and older, protein consumption had no effect on fracture risk. If a high-meat diet reduces fractures, shouldn't it do it in everyone? This is an odd inconsistency, but the study still argues against the low-acid theory, which predicts that a high-protein diet should *increase* fracture risk.
- In the Loma Linda trial, high meat consumption was not the only dietary element that reduced fracture risk. Vegetarians also suffered fewer fractures. "Increasing levels of plant foods decreased wrist fracture risk," with those consuming the most plant foods experiencing "a 68 percent reduction." So *both* vegetarian and high-meat diets reduced fractures. These findings are contradictory and just plain weird. We think this study should be discarded.

In the end, we have three solid fracture trials that argue against low-acid eating. Two show that animal protein reduces fractures. One shows that veganism increases it. One of these studies is retrospective. But the other two are large prospective trials—41,837 and 34,696 participants followed for three and five years. Big numbers. Decent durations. These three studies must be viewed as scientifically sound.

However, many more studies support low-acid eating. They are also more persuasive. In Chapter 7, we summarized five studies showing that, as consumption of animal protein increases, so does fracture risk. Two present worldwide epidemiologic data derived from dozens of studies involving hundreds of thousands of participants:

In addition:

- UCSF researchers documented consumption of animal and plant foods among 1,035 women over sixty-five for seven years. Compared with vegetarians or near-vegetarians, those who ate the most animal foods suffered almost *four times* as many hip fractures.
- Swedish researchers surveyed the protein intake of 39,787 middle-aged adults and then followed them for eleven years. As intake of animal protein increased, so did risk of hip fracture. Among those who consumed the most animal foods, hip fracture risk *doubled*.
- Harvard researchers followed the diets and health of 85,900 women nurses for twelve years. Consumption of "animal protein was associated with an increased risk of fracture."

Of the three nonepidemiological studies, all three are prospective. Compared with the two prospective trials that argue against low-acid eating, all three of the studies bolstering it ran longer—up to four times longer—and one of them had twice as many participants. As a result, the prospective trials supporting low-acid eating are more convincing than the studies that knock it.

Furthermore, in Chapter 7, in the interest of brevity, we did not discuss every study showing that a diet high in fruits and vegetables protects against fractures. Here are two more trials that focus on antioxidant nutrients, which are found *only* in plant foods:

- Swedish scientists surveyed the diets of 66,651 women over forty and followed them for five years. Those who consumed the most vitamin C and E suffered fewer fractures. "An insufficient intake of vitamin E and C may substantially increase risk of hip fracture."

- Utah State researchers identified 1,215 people who'd suffered hip fractures and matched them against 1,349 controls. "Antioxidant intake was associated with reduced risk of osteoporotic hip fractures."

In addition, as we discussed in Chapter 9, six studies show that vitamin K reduces fracture risk, while only one vitamin K report shows no benefit. Small amounts of vitamin K can be obtained from liver, eggs, and beef. But the richest sources are leafy green vegetables. The food that provides the most vitamin K in the American diet is lettuce. So vitamin K levels are a marker for plant foods. The vitamin K trials support low-acid eating.

Finally, also from Chapter 9, one study shows that soy foods reduce fracture risk.

Tallying all the evidence, four studies argue against low-acid eating—the three statistically solid trials that open this chapter and the one from Chapter 9 showing no fracture reduction with vitamin K. Meanwhile, two worldwide epidemiological studies show that animal foods increase fracture risk. Three other studies link animal foods to fractures. Two trials show that antioxidant nutrients found only in fruits and vegetables reduce fracture risk. Six studies show that vitamin K reduces fracture risk. And one shows that soy foods help prevent fractures.

Bottom line: four of eighteen studies (22 percent) contradict the low-acid theory, while fourteen of eighteen (78 percent) support it. The weight of the evidence supports low-acid eating.

Bolstering the case for low-acid eating even more, compared with dairy foods, fruits and vegetables are much more likely to improve bone mineral density. For millions of years, our species evolved eating a largely plant-based diet.

Finally, studies of plant-rich diets—Mediterranean, traditional Asian, vegetarian, vegan, etc.—overwhelming show that a diet high in fruits and vegetables, with a minimum of animal foods, if any, is best for overall health. (See Chapter 7.)

We don't deny the results of the studies that cast doubt on low-acid eating. Life is unpredictable. Every year, the team that wins the

World Series loses about one-third of its games. But it's still the best team—and low-acid eating still offers the most persuasive explanation for osteoporosis.

Protein, Bone Health, and Malnutrition

Some osteoporosis researchers argue against the low-acid theory because it vilifies protein, which, they insist, is essential for strong bones. They have published half a dozen studies arguing that, contrary to the low-acid theory, protein *increases* bone mineral density.

We agree that adequate protein intake is essential for strong bones. The collagen matrix in bone is mostly protein. Our beef, as it were, is not with protein overall but with *animal* protein. As noted earlier, most Americans eat too much of it.

Critics of the low-acid theory assert that bone health often improves when people consume supplements containing meat. They cite studies showing that meat boosts bone mineral density and blood levels of biochemical markers of bone formation.

They're right. Several short-term studies show that increased meat consumption does, indeed, improve measures of bone health. But a closer look at these studies shows that the subjects have been frail nursing home residents over age eighty who are undernourished or malnourished. When people are malnourished, in the short term, their bone health improves with *any* food, vegetable or animal.

Among those over eighty, the digestive tract's ability to digest food declines. Fewer nutrients enter the bloodstream, and many of these people become undernourished or malnourished, which manifests as weight loss and frailty. This is especially true among nursing home residents, particularly those with hip fractures:

- Swiss researchers declare: "Undernutrition and malnutrition increase with advancing age. Patients with hip fracture are often particularly undernourished or malnourished."
- Lithuanian scientists conclude: "Women with osteoporosis had worse appetites and greater malnutrition."

- And Spanish researchers note: "Undernourishment is common in elderly hip fracture patients."

We're persuaded that among malnourished nursing home residents—especially among those recovering from hip fracture—high-protein supplements improve bone health. But we also believe it's a serious mistake to generalize the nutritional needs of frail, malnourished nursing home residents recovering from hip fractures to the general population.

Most Americans are not malnourished. They're *overnourished.* The high-calorie, high-animal-protein diet most Americans eat is a major contributor to the nation's leading health problems.

The researchers who contend that a high-protein/high-meat diet improves bone health have apparently been so preoccupied with the trees that they have lost track of the forest:

- The vast majority of adults are not malnourished frail elders in nursing homes.
- A substantial scientific literature shows that animal foods activate bone-dissolving osteoclasts and suppress bone-building osteoblasts.
- Eighty-five studies show that fruits and vegetables increase bone mineral density, while a mere half dozen trials show that meat boosts BMD.
- Finally, if meat improves bone health in the general population, how do critics of low-acid eating explain all the research showing that a diet high in animal foods increases fracture risk? How do they explain the fact that the countries whose residents consume the most meat and dairy foods have the highest rates of osteoporotic fractures? How do they explain the fact that a high-meat diet activates bone-clearing osteoclasts and suppresses bone-building osteoblasts? How do they explain osteoporosis?

Do Animal Foods Really Increase Calcium Excretion in Urine?

The low-acid theory predicts that high-protein foods should boost the calcium content of urine. Animal foods flood the bloodstream with amino acids unbuffered by the alkaline material in fruits and vegetables. To maintain optimal blood pH, the body must draw acid-neutralizing calcium compounds from bone, which liberate the calcium that winds up in urine.

But critics point to three studies showing that increasing animal protein has no effect on the amount of calcium in urine:

- Researchers at a Veterans Administration hospital in Illinois measured urinary calcium in four men and then fed them a high-meat diet for four months. "There was no change in urinary calcium. High-meat intake does not lead to high levels of calcium in urine and does not induce calcium loss."
- USDA researchers fed fifteen older women a diet with constant calcium (600 milligrams a day), but different amounts of meat (12 percent of calories a day or 20 percent). After eight weeks the two groups showed no differences in urinary calcium. "A high-meat diet did not affect calcium retention or biomarkers of bone metabolism in healthy postmenopausal women."
- University of Saskatchewan researchers measured the urinary calcium in fourteen girls and then fed them moderate or high amounts of the milk protein casein (12 grams or 29 grams). Three hours later "there were no significant differences in calcium excretion."

We don't dispute these results. But many more trials—sixteen—show that as protein consumption increases, the amount of calcium in urine rises. In Chapter 7, we discussed eleven of these studies. Here are the other five:

- Researchers at the University of California, Berkeley, fed six men constant calcium (1,400 milligrams a day) for three months. On a low-protein diet, their urine contained 191milligrams of calcium a day. On a high-protein diet, "urine calcium increased rapidly and significantly" to 277 milligrams a day. "A high-calcium diet is unlikely to prevent a negative calcium balance and bone loss induced by a high-protein diet."

- At the University of Wisconsin–Madison, scientists fed six women a high- or low-protein diet for sixty days and then switched the groups for fifteen days. On the high-protein diet, "urinary calcium approximately doubled."
- University of Connecticut researchers fed adults low- or high-protein diets. "The high-protein diet resulted in hypercalciuria [excess calcium in urine]."
- In Toronto, scientists at St. Michael's Hospital fed twenty middle-aged adults a diet containing 16 or 27 percent of calories from protein. On the high-protein diet, urinary calcium increased significantly.
- Irish researchers fed twenty-four postmenopausal women a moderate-protein diet (70 grams a day) for four weeks and measured their urinary calcium. Then the women ate a high-protein diet (90 grams a day) for four more weeks. On the high-protein diet, urinary calcium increased significantly.

Three of nineteen studies (16 percent) show that a diet high in animal protein has no effect on the amount of calcium in urine. But sixteen of nineteen studies (84 percent) show that, as dietary protein increases, so does urinary calcium—just as the low-acid theory predicts.

Does Excess Calcium in Urine Really Come from Bone?

The low-acid theory says a diet high in animal protein forces the body to take calcium compounds from bone. But some researchers argue that a high-protein diet increases calcium in urine through a *different mechanism.*

They contend that animal protein, especially dairy, stimulates the kidneys to increase calcium filtration, which boosts calcium in urine. In other words, these critics contend, with a high-protein diet extra urinary calcium comes not from bone but from the calcium that animal foods themselves contain, especially dairy foods.

We're happy to concede that some of the extra calcium in urine might come directly from the calcium in animal foods. But again, the scientists who use this finding to question the low-acid theory appear to be fixated on the trees while missing the forest. If the excess calcium in urine does not come from bone, how do they explain the body's regulation of blood pH when a high-protein diet reduces it? How do they explain the many large prospective trials showing that, as intake of animal protein increases, so does risk of fractures? And how do they explain the fact that the countries whose populations consume the most meat and dairy have the highest fracture rates?

If you drink milk and eat cheese and yogurt, some of their calcium might go directly from the gut into the bloodstream and into urine. But this by no means negates the low-acid theory. To our way of thinking, there's only one plausible explanation for the compelling association between diets high in animal foods and high rates of osteoporotic fracture: The body buffers acidic blood by drawing calcium compounds *out of bone.*

The Best Evidence

In medical research, the studies are *never* unanimous. Some trials show that smoking does not cause lung cancer.

This lack of unanimity is not surprising. In life, the evidence rarely points to only one conclusion. Nobel Prize winners sometimes make mistakes. The best restaurants occasionally serve lousy dishes. And the person who wins your heart is never perfect.

We don't deny that a handful of studies contradict the low-acid theory. But with the calcium theory clearly bankrupt, we have a question for skeptics: How do you explain osteoporosis?

We're not arguing that the low-acid theory is flawless, just that the great weight of the evidence supports it—hundreds of studies published worldwide in the peer-reviewed medical literature over the past thirty-plus years. Based on all the evidence, we believe it's the best explanation.

We invite you to examine the evidence yourself. To obtain abstracts of the 1,200-plus studies discussed in this book—the enormous number that support low-acid eating and the few that contest it—see the References at the back of the book.

Evolving Toward Low-Acid Eating—Painlessly

By now you know that bone vitality depends on eating lots of fruits and vegetables, some nuts, and legumes; modest amounts of bread, pasta, and cereal; and not much, if any, meat, poultry, fish, dairy, and eggs. But how much of each?

Going More Alkaline by the Numbers

Starting on page 55, Table 7.1 lists the acidity or alkalinity of only about 120 foods from among the many hundreds we eat. We'd like to see this list expanded to include every food in supermarkets. We hope some researchers get the funding to do this. But even the current abbreviated list provides valuable insights into bone-saving low-acid eating.

Here are the average amounts of acid or alkaline production for the various food groups, ranked from most alkaline to most acid-producing:

Average Acid or Alkaline Effect
− numbers = alkaline
+ numbers = acid producers

Note that the figures for each food group are averages, all based on the same amount—100 grams, or about 3.5 ounces—so you can do a quick at-a-glance comparison of types of foods. Naturally, how much of these foods we actually eat varies, so we've also listed individual foods within these groups, using the typical serving size (in parentheses next to the food). These are the figures you might want to use when examining or planning your own daily diet.

Food Group	3.5-oz. Serving	Typical Serving
Dried fruit	−17.5	
Dried fruit (½ cup)		−9.0
Mixed vegetables	−3.3	
Vegetables (1 cup raw)		−4.0
Vegetables (1 cup cooked)		−6.0
Fruits (excluding juices and dried)	−2.9	
Fruit juice (6 oz.)		−6.0
Fruit (1 cup raw)		−4.0
Fruit (½ cup cooked)		−4.0
Milk and noncheese dairy foods	1.0	
Milk and noncheese dairy (1 cup)		2.5
Yogurt (6 oz.)		2.2
Beans and soy foods	1.1	
Beans (½ cup cooked)		0.6
Soy milk (1 cup)		0.9
Breads, cereals, flours, pastas	6.8	
Wheat or other flour (1 cup)		8.5
Bread (1 slice)		1.7
Pasta (1 cup dry)		2.3
Pasta (1 cup cooked)		0.8
Rice (1 cup dry)		12.0
Rice (1 cup cooked)		2.4
Fish	7.9	
Fish (4 oz. raw)		9.0
Fish (6 oz. cooked)		14.0

Food Group	3.5-oz. Serving	Typical Serving
Cheeses (soft, lower protein content)	8.0	
Soft cheese (2 oz.)		5.0
Eggs	8.2	
Egg (1 egg)		4.0
Meats (including poultry, not fish)	9.4	
Hamburger (3.5-oz. patty)	9.4	
Meat (8-oz. steak or chicken breast)		20.0
Cheeses (hard, higher protein)	23.6	
Hard cheese (2 oz. or 2 slices)		16.0
Grated cheese (1 cup)		24.0

Notice that milk, beans, soy foods, and grain products are acid-producers, but they're much less bone-harming than fish, eggs, meats, and cheeses. It takes only about 1 cup of fruits or vegetables to neutralize one serving of milk, yogurt, beans, bread, pasta, or rice. A plate of pasta (2 cups) topped with 1 to 2 cups of vegetables is neutral or alkaline—and definitely alkaline if accompanied by a side salad or piece of fruit. But if the pasta is smothered in cheese sauce, the dish becomes acid-forming and bone-depleting.

Ounce for ounce, dried fruit is the most alkaline. Regular fruits and vegetables are alkaline, averaging −2.9 and −3.3 respectively. For dried fruit—raisins, prunes, etc.—the average is −17.5. The reason is that fruits and vegetables contain a great deal of water while dried fruits are largely dehydrated, which concentrates their alkalinity.

One type of animal food is substantially more acid-producing than the rest: cheese, for the same reason. Milk, eggs, meats, and fish contain considerable water. Cheese making involves eliminating some of the water in milk, which concentrates the protein. The hard cheeses contain the least water and the most protein per serving, so they are the top acid-formers.

To keep your diet alkaline: It takes about two typical servings of fruits and vegetables to neutralize one small (patty-sized) serving of fish or any other type of meat. For larger portions of meat, such as a sirloin steak or a large chicken breast or thick roast beef sandwich, it will take four typical servings of fruits and vegetables to bring the meal into balance.

And it takes three to four servings of fruits and vegetables to neutralize two sandwich slices of cheese. The cup of cheddar on a small plate of nachos or the cup of mozzarella used on an individual pizza would require five or six servings of fruits and vegetables to neutralize all the acid formed by the cheese.

To put this into perspective consider that a large sausage, egg, and cheese biscuit would need to be balanced by eight servings of fruits or vegetables—one for the egg, two for the two halves of the biscuit, two for the sausage, and three for the cheese. A chicken parmesan submarine sandwich would require a whopping eleven servings of fruits and vegetables to neutralize it: four servings for the sub roll and breading, four servings for the chicken, four servings for the parmesan minus the one alkaline serving of tomato sauce.

A simple option to keep your diet alkaline is to choose a diet built entirely from plant foods making sure to eat more servings of fruits and vegetables than grains and beans.

Alternatively, you can use the following guides to keep your low-acid diet in neutral or alkaline:

- Eat one typical serving of fruits and vegetables for every slice of bread or cup of pasta or rice.
- Eat one-half of a typical serving of fruit or vegetable for each cup of milk, soy milk, yogurt, or beans.
- Eat one typical serving of fruit or vegetable for every egg.
- Eat three to four typical servings for each modest serving of cheese and five to six servings of fruit or vegetables for each large serving of cheese.
- Eat two to three typical servings of fruits and vegetables for each small portion of fish or other meat.
- Eat at least four typical servings of fruits and vegetables for every large (standard American-sized) serving of meat, including poultry.

Cut Down on Meat Easily with Alkaline, Bone-Strengthening Soy Substitutes

Table 7.1 shows that some beans are acid-formers while others are alkaline. Soybeans are somewhat alkaline, while tofu and other soy foods are just about neutral or slightly alkaline. However, a great deal of evidence shows that a diet high in soy foods strengthens bone. It's not clear exactly why. But people who eat lots of soy foods typically use it as a substitute for meat, poultry, and fish, which are much more acid-forming. In addition, people who eat soy foods also tend to eat lots of fruits and vegetables, which are alkaline.

We found thirty-one studies of soy foods' effects on bone:

- Twenty-two (71 percent) show that they improve BMD, decrease urinary calcium excretion, or reduce fracture risk.
- Five (16 percent) are inconclusive.
- Four (13 percent) show no bone benefits.

A sample of the compelling evidence that soy foods strengthen bone:

- Vanderbilt University researchers tracked soy consumption and fractures among 24,403 postmenopausal Chinese women for 4.5 years. As soy intake increased, fracture risk decreased. Compared with those who ate the least soy, women who consumed the most suffered 24 percent fewer fractures.
- Yale researchers fed women identical diets, except for the source of the protein—meat for a while, then soy. While eating the meat, their urine became considerably more acidic.
- Iowa State University researchers fed sixty-nine menopausal women a placebo (3 ounces a day) or soy protein. After six months, bone loss occurred in the placebo group. But in the soy group, BMD increased.
- Japanese researchers measured the urinary calcium of women provided the same diet plus either meat or soy. In the meat

group, urinary calcium excretion increased markedly. But in the soy group, it did not change.

- Hong Kong researchers surveyed the soy intake of 454 postmenopausal Chinese women and then measured their bone mineral density. As soy food consumption increased, so did their BMD.
- Chinese researchers gave ninety women one of three dietary supplements: a placebo, or low or high amounts of soy. After six months, BMD declined in the placebo group but increased in both soy groups, with the greatest increase among those who consumed the high-soy supplement.

One way to incorporate more soy foods into your diet is to eat tofu. Tofu itself is quite bland, but it assumes the flavor of anything it's mixed into. Try it in soups, sauces, and vegetable dishes. For a meatier texture, looked for baked or grilled tofu.

For a meat substitute that looks and tastes similar to lean ground beef, try the soy version. Add soy bits to soups, pasta sauces, lasagna, burritos—anything that calls for ground meat. And try soy substitutes for milk, hot dogs, sausage, chicken, meatballs, and ice cream.

Finally, soy foods contain no saturated fat, so they don't increase the risk of heart disease and many cancers. In fact, an extensive scientific literature shows that soy foods *reduce* the risk of heart disease and breast cancer.

Count Your Daily Fruits and Vegetables

According to the USDA, Americans consume 220 pounds of meat (chicken, turkey, beef, pork, lamb, veal) a year. That's about 10 ounces or 2.5 small servings a day. Bone health requires about three servings of fruits and vegetables to neutralize one serving of meat. So it takes 7.5 daily servings of fruits and vegetables to neutralize the typical American's daily meat intake.

Unfortunately, the average American eats only three daily servings of fruits and vegetables. Worse, one of the nation's most popular vegetables is french fries. Potatoes are quite nutritious—and alkaline (−4.0 per serving). But deep-frying adds so much fat that fries become a nutritional disaster. Eliminate french fries, and the typical American eats fewer than three servings of fruits and vegetables a day.

So meat-eating Americans run an alkaline deficit equivalent to around five servings of fruits and vegetables a day—not counting cheese consumption. No wonder we have an osteoporosis epidemic.

What's "one serving" of fruits and vegetables?

- 1 piece of fruit—1 apple, orange, banana, etc.
- 1 cup of cut-up raw fruit—1 small bowl or 2 handfuls for a typical adult—or ½ cup cooked fruit
- ¾ cup (6 ounces) of 100 percent fruit juice: orange, apple, grape, grapefruit, etc.
- ½ cup dried fruit—a handful of raisins or prunes, etc., for the typical adult
- 1 cup raw or cooked vegetables: peas, carrots, celery, green beans, tomatoes, bell peppers, etc.
- 1 cup leafy greens: lettuce, spinach, chard, etc.

Count your servings every day. It takes only seconds. If you're below five, have a piece of fruit, dried fruit, juice, or a salad or some vegetable soup.

With a little planning, it's easy to get five or more daily servings of fruits and vegetables:

- At breakfast, have juice and/or fruit (1 or 2).
- Midmorning, snack on fruit, dried fruit, or an applesauce cup (1).
- At lunch, have a salad and/or vegetable (1 or 2).
- Midafternoon, snack on fruit or some vegetable strips or chips with salsa (1).
- At dinner, have a salad and/or vegetable (1 or 2).
- Have fruit for dessert (1).

Follow these suggestions and you eat six to nine daily servings of fruits and vegetables. You also save your bones—and reduce your risk of obesity, diabetes, heart disease, and cancer.

A Better Breakfast

If possible, eat breakfast at home. Have fruit juice. If you have cereal, try soy milk instead of cow's milk and add fruit to buffer the grains. If you have toast, instead of butter or cheese, spread on jam or preserves. Have a piece of fruit on the side.

If you eat breakfast on the run or in the car, take fruit and/or vegetables with you.

More Alkaline Lunches and Dinners

Instead of a grilled chicken sandwich and fries, try vegetable soup and a salad. Even if your soup contains meat, dairy, or grain—chicken-noodle or beef-vegetable, etc., you limit acid-producers and eat more plant foods. The same goes for salads. A roast beef sandwich contains one serving of meat (very acid-producing), one or two lettuce leaves (a small amount of alkaline material), and bread (also acid-producing). The result is a sandwich that's bad for bones. A green salad topped with chicken contains one chicken breast (very acid-producing), a heap of lettuce and other vegetables (very alkaline), and no bread. Add a vegetable or fruit and you have a meal that's close to pH-neutral. Or try vegetable fajitas (very alkaline) with pinto beans (slightly acid), tomatoes, and lettuce or avocado (all alkaline) in a wheat tortilla (mildly acid). Skip the cheese and you have a meal that's a delicious bone builder.

A hearty vegetable soup can also be a satisfying dinner. Add some soy meat substitute, and it even tastes meaty. But who has the time or energy to cook a big pot of vegetable soup? If you have just five minutes, you do. See the recipe in Chapter 12 for MC's Soup.

Fruit is often a no-show at dinner. That's easy to change. When melons are in season, add a generous slice to your dinner plate. When it's grapefruit season, have half a grapefruit. Add strawberries, apricots, apples, mangoes, or raspberries to liven up a spinach or lettuce salad. Or serve slices of apples, pears, or bananas.

Bone-Building Snacks and Desserts

Instead of chips or a cookie, have fruit. Fruit easily slips into a backpack or desk drawer so it's handy when you feel a hunger pang.

Among rated fruits, raisins are among the most alkaline, coming in at −21.0. Ounce for ounce, that's almost four times more alkaline than the most alkaline nondried fruit, bananas (−5.5), and considerably more alkaline than the most alkaline vegetable, spinach (−14.0). As a result, raisins might be viewed as bone-strengthening "pills."

Raisins and other dried fruits—figs, apples, apricots, banana chips, mangoes, and prunes (dried plums)—can satisfy a sweet tooth. They are easily portable and keep for a long time without refrigeration. Carry snack-size boxes of raisins with you and enjoy them anytime, anywhere.

Breads are acid-producing, but add a few raisins, and raisin bread becomes alkaline. Or use raisins or other dried fruits in cooking. At breakfast, added to cereal, they tip the balance toward alkaline and save your bones.

Dentists often discourage dried fruit because they are high in sugar and sticky, which may increase risk of tooth decay and gum disease. To eliminate the stickiness, store dried fruit in water. The fruit becomes slightly rehydrated and much less sticky.

If you have access to a microwave, instead of coffee or tea, try a quick cup of vegetable soup. Small soup boxes can be kept unrefrigerated in a locker, backpack, or desk drawer.

Eating Out the Low-Acid Way

Forty years ago, Mom packed the kids off to school with a bag lunch (including a piece of fruit) and cooked dinner from scratch, often with both a salad and a vegetable. Today, most mothers work outside the home. Parents have long commutes. Kids have hectic schedules. More than half of meals are eaten away from home. And many families rarely have family dinners. For millions of Americans, home cooking has been replaced by fast food.

In 1970, Americans spent $6 billion on fast food. By 2000, the figure was $110 billion. Every day one-quarter of the U.S. adult population visits a fast-food restaurant. In 1975, three-quarters of U.S. food dollars were spent on items prepared at home. Today, half of U.S. food dollars are spent at restaurants, mostly fast-food places. McDonald's is the nation's largest purchaser of beef, pork, and potatoes. The typical American consumes three fast-food burgers a week.

McDonald's, Burger King, Wendy's, Arby's, KFC—fast-food outlets sell mostly high-fat animal products that rot your bones and boost your risk of heart disease and cancer. But even in these nutritional deserts there are oases of alkaline items. Most fast-food places serve salads. Many of them include animal foods—chicken, bacon, cheese, etc.—but the salads are more alkaline (and if you don't eat the cheese, lower in saturated fat) than the other menu items.

A Big Mac contains 25 grams of animal protein. A McDonald's Southwest Chicken Salad contains 30 grams of protein. These are bone-killing meals—and high in calories and fat. But opt for a Southwest Salad without the chicken and you get no animal protein and just 6 grams of vegetable protein, which is well buffered by all the vegetable ingredients. A no-chicken Southwest Salad is also low in calories and fat. Top off your no-chicken Southwest Salad with a Fruit and Walnut Salad and you get 4 grams of vegetable protein well buffered by lots of alkaline, bone-building fruit.

Other fast-food places also offer salads. Burger King features Veggie Burgers. Taco Bell has bean burritos—ask for less cheese or none and extra lettuce and tomatoes. Wendy's offers baked potatoes. You can get them topped with broccoli. And if you like Middle Eastern food, a falafel sandwich stuffed with cucumber, lettuce, and tomato is tasty and filling yet contains no animal protein at all.

If you can eat bone-building meals at McDonald's and Burger King, you can eat them anywhere. Most restaurants have vegetarian entree options. Salads are available everywhere. Consider making a meal of soup and salad. Or scan the side dishes for vegetable items. Asian cuisines often combine small amounts of animal food with generous amounts of vegetables. And if you keep some fruit or a box of raisins handy, you can buffer the animal protein you consume—and keep your bones strong and fracture-resistant.

Menu Planning for One Week of Low-Acid Eating

Planning for low-acid eating is easy. There are only two rules: Avoid or limit meats, eggs, cheese, and other dairy foods. Include two servings of vegetable and/or fruit at every meal.

Seven Bone-Building Breakfasts

Dishes that begin with capital letters are recipes in Chapter 12.

Breakfast 1: A bowl of fruit (cherries, apricots, nectarines, berries) or a Fruit Smoothie; toast with peanut butter, avocado, Nutella, or fruit jam or spread

Breakfast 2: Oatmeal cooked with apples and raisins; a glass of juice

Breakfast 3: Updated Southern Breakfast: Yellow Corn Grits, Sautéed Greens, and Fresh Tomato; tempeh bacon

Breakfast 4: Scrambled Tofu with Vegetables; oven-roasted breakfast potatoes

Breakfast 5: Vegetarian English breakfast—small portions of toast, baked beans, hash browns, grilled tomatoes, and onions; glass of juice

Breakfast 6: Cold cereal topped with strawberries and soy milk; banana

Breakfast 7: Berry pancakes topped with applesauce or raspberry sauce; veggie sausage

Or come up with your own low-acid breakfast by putting together combinations from the lists that follow.

Choose at least one of the following:

- Fresh or frozen fruit
- Fruit juice or fruit smoothie
- Canned or cooked fruit or fruit sauce
- Vegetables—tomato, potato, mushrooms, spinach, avocado, or other greens
- Scrambled tofu or soy milk

Choose one of the following:

- Toast
- Cereal
- Hot or cold cereal
- Pancakes
- Grits

Add no more than one of the following if you like:

- Veggie sausage
- Tempeh bacon
- Nutella, honey, jam, fruit spread
- Muffin
- Beans

Avoid or use very sparingly:

- Eggs
- Cheese or cream cheese
- Breakfast meats
- Croissants

Seven Luscious Lunches

Lunch 1: MC's Soup, wheat roll, piece of fruit

Lunch 2: Falafel pita sandwich with cucumber, lettuce, tomato; watermelon

Lunch 3: Mediterranean Potato Salad; spinach salad with fruit

Lunch 4: Red Pepper Hummus wrap with grated carrots and tomato; cut-up fruit
Lunch 5: Vegetarian chili; green salad; sorbet with raspberries
Lunch 6: Eggless Salad Sandwich; tomato basil salad
Lunch 7: Thai noodle soup with spinach, mushrooms, and corn; carrots and bean dip; berries

Vegetable and bean-vegetable soups make great lunches. So do hearty grain- or bean-based salads with vegetables, such as black bean and corn salad with red peppers. Sandwiches and wraps chock full of vegetables are easy to store and carry. Good sandwich/wrap vegetables include spinach, tomatoes, cucumbers, carrots, peppers, and avocados. Or try hummus and black bean or white bean spread. Include at least two servings of fruit and vegetables paired with at least one serving of either a grain or a bean or both.

Seven Spectacular Suppers

The options for making delicious low-acid meals for supper are nearly endless:

Supper 1: Triple-Vegetable Pasta Primavera; cucumber, avocado, tomato salad; lemon sorbet with Berry Sauce
Supper 2: Vegetable Fajita Burrito; mashed sweet potato; corn; cut-up fruit
Supper 3: Roasted portobello mushrooms and red peppers on a bed of quinoa; steamed artichoke; Cabbage and Fruit Salad; Strawberry-Rhubarb Crumble
Supper 4: Curried Potatoes and Peas; Coconut Dahl; mango chutney; fruit salad
Supper 5: Grilled tofu, zucchini, asparagus, and mushrooms; corn on the cob; Cretan Salad
Supper 6: Thai Red Curry with Vegetables; Sweet and Spicy Potatoes and Kale; cucumber salad; mango
Supper 7: Roasted root vegetables; Summer Ratatouille with Polenta; baked apple stuffed with raisins

Of course, lunch ideas can be used to create delicious suppers, and vice versa. Just include at least one vegetable and one fruit for supper. Add a starchy vegetable, bean, or grain and you'll have a hearty, well-balanced, bone-building meal.

Shifting Kids' Diets Toward Low-Acid Eating

If kids eat a low-acid diet, plant foods can supply all the calcium and "mortar" nutrients they need. The issue is not how to get enough calcium without milk. It's how to get kids to eat the fruits and vegetables they should—not only for strong bones but also for overall health.

Many kids like fruit more than they like vegetables. So give them lots of fruit:

- *Any* fruit helps build strong bones—fresh, canned, dried, or frozen. You might prefer fresh fruit, but if your kids enjoy canned peaches or fruit cocktail, that's fine.
- Reduce or eliminate chips, cookies, and other junk snacks from your pantry. Position a fruit bowl prominently in your kitchen and keep it filled with fresh fruit in season. The more kids see fruit, the more likely they are to eat it. Keep a fruit bowl near your television too.
- Serve fruit at every meal. Kids may ignore a fruit bowl, especially when eating the fruit involves any work. But if you core and slice apples, slice melons, or peel oranges, bananas, tangerines, or a pineapple, and put them in front of kids, they're usually happy to eat them.
- Buy raisins in snack-size boxes. Send raisin boxes with kids to school and activities.
- Applesauce and fruit cups are available in single-serving containers. Keep a supply on hand to tuck into lunch boxes or children's backpacks. Applesauce or apple-berry sauces also

make a tasty dip for graham crackers and a delicious topping for pancakes.

- Instead of serving milk at meals, serve smoothies (see the next chapter).
- For a quick, tasty, nutritious, bone-building snack, peel bananas, insert Popsicle sticks into one end, and freeze them. Presto: frozen bananas.
- Splurge on out-of-the-ordinary fruits: kiwis, mangoes, blueberries, blackberries, raspberries, and melons. Some kids who turn up their noses at apples, oranges, and bananas are happy to eat more exotic fruits. Many kids list berries and melons among their favorite foods.
- Serve fruit for dessert. Or try a fruit-filled pie or crisp: apple, cherry, berry, etc. Pies are higher in fat than plain fruit and more acid-forming because of the flour and butter in the crust. But a slice of blueberry pie is considerably more bone building than a piece of any cake.
- Experiment with chutneys. Mango and other chutneys pair beautifully with many vegetable dishes. Pineapple salsa is a delicious addition to Mexican or other spicy cuisines.
- Add fruit to savory dishes. Raisins, figs, prunes, apricots, and other fruits can be included in many dishes. Try pineapple chunks on pizza. Slices of apples, pears, strawberries, and other fruits can be added to salads. And try a handful of raisins in spaghetti sauce.
- Children learn from observing their parents. If you eat a low-acid diet, they just might, too.
- Encourage kids to have fun experiences that involve fruits and vegetables. Take them to U-pick-it farms or farmers' markets or grow some fruits and vegetables at home. Most kids love picking strawberries and other fruits.
- Spend time with kids in the kitchen. Children often show more interest in healthful eating when they're involved in preparing food. Even small children can wash fruits and vegetables, add

continued

ingredients to mixing bowls, and stir. Older children can be introduced to knife skills, recipes, and making salads or other dishes.

Some kids enjoy a wide range of vegetables, while others are finicky. Here are some ways to overcome kids' veggie phobias:

- Serve a vegetable first when kids are hungriest. It doesn't have to be anything fancy. Try carrot and celery sticks, cherry or grape tomatoes, or blanched green beans or broccoli florets.
- Many children love dips. Try offering baby carrots, cucumber slices, or celery sticks with hummus (see the recipe in the next chapter), salsa, salad dressing, or even peanut butter.
- The one vegetable most kids love is french fries, a nutritional loser. Instead, cut potatoes into strips and bake them. Roasted potato strips look similar to fries and have the same crunch—but they're more nutritious.
- Tomato-based spaghetti sauce is another kid favorite. For picky eaters, hide other vegetables in the sauce: chopped onions, grated carrots, and diced broccoli or greens. Soups are another great place to slip in extra vegetables. Wraps also work well.
- Sandwiches and wraps can also include extra vegetables: a few spinach leaves, thinly sliced cucumbers or tomatoes, or mashed avocado.
- Many children love pasta. By itself, pasta is acid-forming. But add some vegetables and it becomes a bone builder.

Recipes for Low-Acid Eating

Low-acid eating is easy and delicious. Try these tasty and straightforward recipes on their own or use the meals plans outlined in Chapter 11. Think of these as a starting place. You may also want to experiment with deacidifying your family favorites—by taking out or reducing the amount of meat and cheese and increasing the vegetable amounts. Sometimes beans or tofu or tempeh can be substituted for the meat and a nondairy milk or other product can be substituted for the dairy ingredients. And, of course, there are lots of recipe resources on the Web and in vegetarian and vegan cookbooks as well as heart-healthy and cancer-prevention ones for increasing your daily servings of fruit and vegetables. Enjoy.

Fruit Smoothies

Serves 2

These luscious smoothies can be served as a beverage or dessert.

1. Berry
2 cups frozen berries
1 to 2 tablespoons maple syrup
2 tablespoons calcium-fortified orange juice
½ to 1 cup water or soy milk as needed

Place the berries, maple syrup, and orange juice in a blender and blend until smooth, stirring and adding water or soy milk as needed to achieve the desired thickness.

2. Tropical
1 cup banana chunks, frozen
1 cup pineapple pieces
½ cup unsweetened apple juice, or more if desired

Place the banana chunks and pineapple pieces in a blender with the apple juice. Blend, stopping occasionally to move unblended fruit toward the blades. For a thinner smoothie, add more juice. Serve immediately.

Updated Southern Breakfast: Yellow Corn Grits, Sautéed Greens, and Fresh Tomato

Serves 2 or 3

3 cups water, or more if needed
1 cup organic yellow grits
2 teaspoons Bragg's Liquid Aminos or soy sauce
Freshly ground black pepper to taste
¾ cup chopped sweet onion
6 cremini or button mushrooms, quartered
1 teaspoon balsamic vinegar
3 cups chopped raw greens: kale, braising greens, bok choy, chard, etc.
1 to 2 ripe fresh tomatoes, cut into bite-sized chunks
Hot sauce to taste

Boil the water in a medium saucepan, add the grits, and stir. Reduce the heat to simmer, stirring occasionally, until the water is absorbed, about 10 minutes. Add more water if needed to bring the grits to the desired consistency. Stir in 1 teaspoon of the Bragg's Liquid Aminos (or soy sauce) and black pepper.

While the grits are cooking, sauté the onion and mushrooms with the remaining teaspoon of Bragg's Liquid Aminos (or soy sauce) and the vinegar until the onion begins to soften and the mushrooms start to release their juices, about 3 minutes. Add the greens and sauté for 3 to 5 minutes, until the greens are wilted.

Serve the grits and greens with the chopped tomatoes and hot sauce.

Scrambled Tofu with Vegetables

Serves 4

This nutritious scramble is great with roasted breakfast potatoes. Or wrap it in a whole wheat tortilla for a delicious breakfast burrito.

1 teaspoon vegetable oil
½ cup chopped sweet onion
1 medium carrot, grated
½ red bell pepper, finely chopped
4 button mushrooms, sliced
½ pound firm tofu, crumbled
¼ teaspoon ground turmeric
¼ teaspoon ground cumin
⅛ teaspoon freshly ground black pepper
2 teaspoons soy sauce

Heat the oil in a nonstick skillet over medium heat. Add the onion, carrot, bell pepper, and mushrooms and cook, stirring often, for 3 minutes. Add the tofu, turmeric, cumin, black pepper, and soy sauce. Cook, stirring gently, for 3 to 5 minutes and serve immediately.

MC's Soup

Serves 2 to 4

The ingredients require no preparation at all. Just throw everything into a soup pot and heat.

1 32-ounce container of any type of vegetable soup: broccoli, tomato, carrot, mushroom, sweet corn, butternut squash, black bean, French onion, carrot/ginger, red pepper/tomato, or curried red lentil, available at health food stores and many supermarkets (visit imaginefoods.com or pacificfoods.com)
1 10-ounce package of frozen vegetables, or, if you have time, 3 to 4 cups peeled (if necessary) and chopped fresh vegetables (such as zucchini, carrots, mushrooms, spinach, or green beans)
1 cup mild, medium, or spicy tomato salsa
1 cup chopped tofu or soy ground beef substitute (optional)
1 15-ounce can kidney, garbanzo, pinto, or other beans, drained (optional)

Mix everything in a soup pot. Heat and eat. This soup is hearty enough for a meal. Refrigerated, it keeps for several days. If you have access to a microwave, it's great for lunch at work.

Mediterranean Potato Salad

Serves 6

5 or 6 medium new potatoes, cut into bite-sized pieces
1 yellow or red onion, slivered
1 red bell pepper, cut into thin 2-inch-long strips
2 tablespoons plus 1 teaspoon olive oil
2 tablespoons balsamic vinegar
20 green beans, snapped into 1-inch pieces
2 small celery stalks, tops removed, diced
1 tablespoon minced fresh oregano or other fresh herbs
1 teaspoon Dijon mustard
Salt and freshly ground pepper to taste

Cover the potatoes with water in a saucepan. Boil until just soft when pierced with a fork, about 15 to 20 minutes. Drain. Transfer to a medium bowl and set aside.

Sauté the onion and bell pepper in 1 teaspoon of the olive oil and 1 tablespoon of the balsamic vinegar until soft, about 5 minutes. Add the vegetables to the cooling potatoes.

Bring a small pot of water to a boil, add the green beans, and boil for 3 to 4 minutes, until crisp-tender and still bright green. Drain and add the green beans to the bowl. Then add the celery and fresh herbs to the vegetable mixture. Mix the remaining 2 tablespoons of olive oil with the mustard and the remaining 1 tablespoon vinegar (you may use red wine vinegar here instead of balsamic if you prefer) in a small container with a lid. Shake to mix. Pour the dressing over the potato mixture, add salt and black pepper, and stir. Refrigerate until chilled. Stir again before serving.

Eggless Salad Sandwich

Makes 4 sandwiches

This salad has the flavor and appearance of egg salad without the saturated fat or animal protein.

½ 16-ounce package firm reduced-fat tofu, drained and mashed (1 cup)
1 scallion, both white and green parts or ¼ small sweet onion, finely chopped
1 celery stalk, finely chopped
1 tablespoon sweet pickle relish
2 tablespoons vegan mayonnaise or other eggless mayonnaise
2 teaspoons stone-ground mustard
2 teaspoons reduced-sodium soy sauce
¼ teaspoon each ground cumin, ground turmeric, and garlic powder (or ½ teaspoon curry powder)
8 slices whole-grain bread
4 lettuce leaves
8 tomato slices

Mix the mashed tofu with the scallion, celery, relish, mayo, mustard, soy sauce, cumin, turmeric, and garlic powder. Mix.

Spread on whole-grain bread, add lettuce and tomato, and top with another slice of bread.

Red Pepper Hummus

Makes 2 cups

1 15-ounce can garbanzo beans
½ cup water-packed roasted red pepper
3 tablespoons fresh lemon juice
1 tablespoon tahini (sesame seed butter)
1 garlic clove, peeled
¼ teaspoon ground cumin

Drain the garbanzo beans. Place in a food processor or blender with the roasted peppers, lemon juice, tahini, garlic, and cumin. Process until very smooth, 1 to 2 minutes.

Triple-Vegetable Pasta Primavera

Serves 4 to 6

8 ounces dried pasta, any shape
1 medium yellow onion, chopped
4 garlic cloves, minced
8 ounces cremini mushrooms, quartered
2 tablespoons olive oil or trans-fat-free margarine
1 tablespoon flour
2 tablespoons water
1 cup soy milk
Salt and freshly ground black pepper to taste
Hot red pepper flakes to taste (optional)
3 carrots, sliced
2 cups bite-sized broccoli florets
2 cups snap peas, tips trimmed, cut in half
1 pint cherry tomatoes
½ cup chopped fresh basil leaves

Boil the pasta in salted water until done. Drain and set aside.

Sauté the onion, garlic, and mushrooms in the olive oil in a skillet or sauté pan over medium heat until soft, about 5 to 6 minutes. Mix the flour and water together until smooth. Add to the mushroom and onion mixture and stir. Add the soy milk and stir over low heat until the mixture thickens, about 3 minutes. Add the salt and pepper and red pepper flakes, turn off the heat, and set aside.

Steam the carrots in a small amount of water for about 5 minutes. Add the broccoli and cook for 3 minutes. Add the snap peas and cook for 2 to 3 minutes. Drain. In a large bowl, toss the pasta with the mushroom sauce. Add the steamed vegetables and stir, over low heat if necessary to reheat.

Top with cherry tomatoes and basil leaves and serve.

Berry Sauce

Serves 6 as a dessert topping

1½ cups frozen raspberries
¼ cup orange juice
1 cup fresh or frozen blueberries

Combine the raspberries and orange juice in a small saucepan. Simmer until the raspberries become saucelike, about 5 minutes. Add the blueberries and cook for 2 more minutes. Serve warm over fruit sorbet, poached pears, or vanilla nondairy ice cream. Leftover sauce keeps in the refrigerator for a week and can be used on cereal or oatmeal.

Vegetable Fajita Burrito

Serves 2

These burritos are delicious served with green salad or mashed sweet potatoes. If you like, garnish them with avocado and/or chopped fresh cilantro and additional salsa.

1 cup canned refried beans
¾ cup fresh salsa
½ teaspoon ground cumin
1 cup yellow or white corn kernels, fresh or frozen

3 cups chopped vegetables: any combination of onion, red and green bell peppers, mushrooms, zucchini, yellow squash, etc.
1 teaspoon vegetable oil
½ teaspoon chili powder or other spicy seasoning mix
2 10-inch or larger flour tortillas, white or whole wheat

Heat the refried beans in a small pan and stir in ¼ cup of the salsa and the cumin. Steam the corn until just cooked. Sauté the vegetable mixture in the oil in a large skillet over high heat until sizzling. Add the chili powder or other spices. Warm the tortillas on a dry flat pan. To assemble the burritos, spread half of the beans on each tortilla, add half of the vegetable mixture and half of the corn, and top each with ¼ cup of salsa. Wrap up the burrito by starting to roll the tortilla and then folding in the sides before completing the rolling.

Cabbage and Fruit Salad

Serves 4 to 6

Delicious cold or at room temperature.

1 small Napa cabbage or ½ small head green or red cabbage, diced (about 4 cups)
½ large English cucumber, chopped
1 large carrot, grated
½ teaspoon peeled and grated fresh ginger or ¼ teaspoon ground ginger
¼ cup rice vinegar
Freshly ground black pepper
1 ripe mango, peeled and cut into small pieces, or ¼ cup sliced dried apricots
1 firm avocado, peeled, pitted, and cut into small pieces (optional)
¼ cup chopped raw cashews

Toss the cabbage, cucumber, carrot, and ginger with the vinegar and black pepper. Cover and let sit until ready to serve. Add the fruit, avocado, and cashews. Toss and serve.

Strawberry-Rhubarb Crumble

Makes 1 9-inch square pan

2 pints fresh strawberries
2 or 3 large stalks rhubarb
1 tablespoon sugar or maple syrup
1 teaspoon ground cinnamon
1 cup rolled oats
¼ cup whole wheat or other flour
¼ cup brown sugar
¼ cup margarine trans-fat-free or vegetable oil

Preheat the oven to 350°F. Hull the strawberries and cut them in half. Chop the rhubarb into bite-sized pieces. Toss together with 1 tablespoon sugar and ½ teaspoon of the cinnamon in a 9-inch square pan. Mix the remaining ingredients, including the remaining ½ teaspoon cinnamon, in a small bowl to make a crumble topping. Sprinkle the topping over the fruit and bake for 30 to 40 minutes, until bubbly. Serve warm or room temperature.

Curried Potatoes and Peas

Serves 4

1 medium yellow onion, chopped
1 teaspoon minced garlic (optional)
1 tablespoon vegetable oil
4 medium white or red potatoes, cut into ½-inch pieces
3 carrots, halved lengthwise and sliced into half moons
1 to 2 cups bite-sized cauliflower florets (optional)
1 cup water, or more as needed
1 to 2 teaspoons soy sauce
2 cups fresh or frozen peas
1 teaspoon curry powder
Chopped tomato, chopped fresh cilantro, and/or mango chutney for garnish (optional)

In a large skillet or sauté pan over medium heat, sauté the onion and the garlic (if using) in the oil until they begin to brown, about 2 to 3 minutes. Add the potatoes, carrots, and cauliflower (if using). Cook and stir for 3 minutes. Add the water and soy sauce to the pan and stir. Cover, reduce heat to low, and simmer for 5 to 7 minutes. If the water dries up before the vegetables soften, add more. When the carrots are nearly soft, add the peas and curry powder. Cook, uncovered, until most of the water has evaporated. Cover and keep warm until ready to serve. Serve with any or all of the suggested garnishes.

Cretan Salad

Serves 4 as a side dish or 2 as an entree

You can serve this on a bed of greens if you like.

4 ripe fresh tomatoes, quartered and then sliced
½ large English cucumber, peeled, quartered lengthwise, and sliced
1 large avocado, peeled, pitted, and cut into bite-sized pieces
1 red bell pepper, cut into bite-sized pieces
½ cup fresh basil leaves
1 to 2 tablespoons olive oil
3 tablespoons balsamic vinegar
Freshly cracked black pepper to taste
¼ cup shelled salted pistachio nuts

Put the tomatoes, cucumber, avocado, and red pepper in a bowl. Add the basil leaves, dress with olive oil and balsamic vinegar, and sprinkle with black pepper and pistachio nuts. Serve cold or at room temperature.

Coconut Dahl

Serves 4

3 cups water
1 cup dry red or orange lentils
1 cup chopped yellow onion

1 cup quartered cremini mushrooms
½ teaspoon cumin
½ teaspoon garam marsala
1 cup lite coconut milk
3 cups fresh spinach leaves
1 tablespoon balsamic vinegar
Salt and pepper, to taste

Bring 3 cups of water to a boil. Rinse lentils and add them to the boiling water. Add onion and allow mixture to simmer uncovered until the lentils soften, about 15 minutes. Add more water if needed to keep lentils moist. Add mushrooms, cumin, garam marsala, and coconut milk. Simmer uncovered another 5 minutes. Add spinach leaves, vinegar, and season with salt and pepper. If a thicker mixture is desired, continue cooking until desired consistency is achieved. Keep warm until ready to serve.

Thai Red Curry with Vegetables

Serves 6

4 carrots, sliced
4 medium red potatoes, cut into bite-sized pieces
2 teaspoons of Thai red curry paste, more if additional heat is desired
2 teaspoons of canola oil
1 12-ounce can of lite coconut milk
2 cups green beans, tips removed, cut into 1-inch pieces
1 cup halved button mushrooms
1 15-ounce can baby corn, drained
1 cup broccoli florets
1 tablespoon soy sauce
1 teaspoon sugar, agave nectar, or other sweetener
1 tablespoon fresh lime juice
1 cup firm tofu, cubed (optional)
Sliced cherry tomatoes and cilantro for garnish (optional)

In a large wok or pot, steam carrots and potatoes in 1 inch of water until starting to soften, about 10 minutes. Drain water off and add curry paste and canola oil. Stir mixture over medium heat until well blended. Add coconut milk and remaining vegetables. Simmer for 10 minutes. Add soy sauce, sugar, lime juice, and tofu, if using. Warm over low heat for another 5 minutes. Serve hot in a bowl by itself or with rice. Garnish with sliced cherry tomatoes and cilantro, if desired.

Sweet and Spicy Potatoes and Kale

Serves 6

2 small or 1 large garnet yam or sweet potato, cut into bite-sized chunks
1 onion, sliced into rings and the rings quartered
2 large garlic cloves, minced
1 tablespoon maple syrup
1 tablespoon vegetarian Worcestershire sauce (optional)
½ to 1 teaspoon Thai chili paste, to taste
1 bunch kale, stems stripped away and leaves chopped (about 4 cups)
½ lemon

Put the yams or sweet potatoes in a deep skillet and barely cover them with water. Cover the skillet and boil the yams or sweet potatoes for 5 to 10 minutes, until soft when pierced with a fork. Add onion and garlic and simmer until half the water has boiled away. Add the maple syrup, Worcestershire sauce (if using), chili paste, and kale. Simmer until the kale is soft, about 10 minutes. Squeeze the lemon over the mixture and serve.

Summer Ratatouille with Polenta

Serves 8 to 10

2 small eggplants
2 medium zucchini
2 medium yellow squash

2 red bell peppers
1 tablespoon olive oil (2 tablespoons if roasting the vegetables)
¼ cup balsamic vinegar
1 large or 2 small yellow onions, finely chopped
4 celery stalks, chopped
4 to 6 garlic cloves, finely chopped
½ cup vegetable broth or water
4 fresh Roma (plum) tomatoes, chopped
1 12-ounce can crushed tomatoes
About 1 tablespoon soy sauce or sea salt to taste
Baked Polenta (recipe follows), 10 cups cooked brown rice, or 10 cups whole-grain pasta
¼ cup chopped fresh herbs, such as basil, oregano, thyme, and chives

To grill: Light a charcoal or gas grill. Trim off the stems and thickly slice the eggplants. Trim off the ends and slice the zucchini and squash lengthwise. Cut the red peppers in half and remove the seeds and core. Grill over high heat until the vegetables are browned. Allow to cool. Cut the grilled vegetables into bite-sized pieces.

To roast: Preheat the oven to 400°F. Trim the eggplants and cut into bite-sized pieces. Core and seed the red peppers and cut into bite-sized pieces. Trim off the ends and cut the zucchini and squash into bite-sized pieces. Spread the cut vegetables in flat pans and drizzle with 1 tablespoon of the olive oil and 2 tablespoons of the vinegar. Roast the vegetables for 20 to 30 minutes, until they begin to brown on the edges.

Put 1 tablespoon olive oil in a large, heavy pot over medium-high heat, add the onion, celery, and garlic, and sauté until browned, about 5 minutes, adding 1 tablespoon of the remaining balsamic vinegar as the celery and onion begin to soften. Once the onions have browned, add the broth or water and turn the heat down to simmer.

Add the grilled vegetables, Roma tomatoes, and canned tomatoes. Simmer for about 15 minutes, until all the vegetables are cooked.

Add the soy sauce or salt to taste. Serve over polenta, rice, or pasta and top with fresh herbs.

Baked Polenta

Serves 8

6 to 7 cups water
2 cups white or yellow coarsely ground cornmeal
2 teaspoons Bragg's Liquid Aminos or soy sauce
1 teaspoon olive oil

Boil the water in a saucepan. Add the cornmeal and stir well. Simmer the cornmeal until the mixture is oatmeal consistency and no longer crunchy (time will vary depending on the coarseness of the cornmeal). Follow the package directions.

Scoop the cooked polenta (cornmeal) into a pie plate greased with ½ teaspoon of the olive oil. Drizzle the remaining ½ teaspoon of olive oil over the top. Cover and refrigerate for later use or put into a preheated 450°F oven and bake for 30 to 40 minutes, until the polenta begins to brown. Remove from the oven and divide into 8 portions for serving.

Top with Summer Ratatouille, sautéed mushrooms, or grilled vegetables and serve hot.

As Important as Low-Acid Eating: Walk Your Way to Stronger Bones

BEYOND LOW-ACID EATING, the single best bone strengthener is exercise. But you *don't* have to join a gym, sweat buckets, or get your heart rate into the aerobic range. All that's necessary is a daily thirty- to sixty-minute walk or equivalent exercise. Really. That's all it takes.

We found sixty-eight studies published since 1975 that correlate physical activity and fracture risk:

- Fifty-nine (87 percent) show that regular, moderate exercise (walking, gardening, dancing, golf, etc.) provides substantial protection against fractures.
- Nine (13 percent) show that exercise has no effect on fracture risk.

The evidence is overwhelmingly in favor of regular, moderate exercise for fracture prevention—not to mention that exercise also helps control weight and reduces risk of constipation, hemorrhoids, insomnia, diabetes, anxiety problems, high cholesterol, high blood pressure, heart disease, Alzheimer's, and many cancers.

Exercise reduces risk of fractures for two reasons: It strengthens bone. And it improves balance, which reduces risk of falling, the trigger for the vast majority of osteoporotic fractures.

Modest Activity, Major Bone Benefits

The research speaks for itself. A few of the many studies:

- Finnish scientists surveyed physical activity in 3,262 middle-aged men and then followed them for twenty-one years. Compared with those who were most sedentary, the most active men suffered a whopping 62 percent fewer hip fractures.
- Harvard researchers tracked walking and other exercise among 61,200 U.S. female nurses for twelve years. As time spent walking, dancing, gardening, etc., increased, their hip fracture risk steadily decreased. Exercise for an hour a day and you cut risk of hip fracture in half.
- In a six-year trial of 14,015 nurses, Danish scientists found that regular exercise reduces hip fracture risk 50 percent.
- French scientists asked 6,901 older women how they spent their time and asked them again almost four years later. Regular moderate exercise reduced hip fractures by 50 percent.
- Norwegian researchers surveyed exercise and fractures in 12,270 middle-aged adults and then resurveyed them seven years later. Compared with the least active, those who were most active suffered 40 percent fewer fractures.

All five of these trials are prospective. The numbers are large, averaging 19,530 participants. And the durations are long, averaging ten years. Meanwhile, the participants were not athletes. They were ordinary people, middle-aged or older, who walked, gardened, danced, did housework, and played tennis or engaged in similar activities. Nonetheless, the results are compelling. Modest physical activity—the equivalent of brisk walking for thirty to sixty minutes a day—reduced hip fractures by half.

Exercise Around the World

So far we've attributed the fact that the countries with the highest calcium intake suffer the most fractures to the consumption of animal foods. But that's not the only reason. The countries with the most fractures are the affluent nations, where most people work in office jobs, where most adults have cars, where there's mass transit. In the developing nations, where fracture rates are lower, people walk more.

Which is more important—low-acid eating or exercise? Both are crucial. The osteoporosis cure stands on two legs: low-acid eating and regular, moderate exercise.

The Best Exercise for Fracture Prevention

Not all exercise strengthens bone. To reduce fracture risk, it must be *weight-bearing*. Your bones must support your weight—as they do when you walk, run, dance, garden, or do housework. Activities that are not weight-bearing—swimming and cycling, for example—are great fun and have many health benefits. But they do not reduce fracture risk.

Weight-bearing exercise helps prevent fractures at any age. While most studies have targeted middle-aged or older people, several have correlated exercise and fractures among adolescents and young adults. In young girls and boys, in teenagers, and in young adult military recruits, regular, moderate activity reduces fracture risk significantly (see the last section in this chapter).

Walking puts weight on the legs and spine. It helps prevent hip and vertebral fractures. But what about arm and wrist fractures? Effective approaches include gardening, which involves carrying things, and the yoga poses that put weight on the wrist and arms. You can also carry light weights, such as canned foods, while you walk or lift weight, including unloading groceries or a dishwasher.

How Weight-Bearing Exercise Strengthens Bone

Bones are similar to muscles. Use muscles, and they become bigger and stronger. Stop using them, and they weaken and atrophy. Like muscles, when bones are used—when they support weight or carry a load (within reason)—they get stronger.

When we use our muscles, they develop microtears. We repair these tears by creating new muscle tissue—and more of it—which is why sustained exercise produces bigger, bulkier muscles.

Similarly, when our bones bear weight, they experience strain. Strain produces microscopic weak spots. As those weak spots develop, the bone cells in the vicinity release chemicals that signal the body: Weak spot! Send help! Bone-clearing osteoclasts converge on the problem area and dissolve the weakened bone. Then osteoblasts migrate from nearby bone marrow, enter the tiny breach, and create new bone. Normal strain stimulates the creation of new, strong, robust bone. In other words, weight-bearing activities give bones a reason to thrive.

In the absence of normal strain, when bones don't support weight or contend with the torque and impact of activities like walking, very little new bone is created. Old bone slowly weakens and over time becomes prone to fracture. Consider early space travel. While weightless in space, astronauts of the 1970s did not experience normal bone strain. Their bones weakened, which caused problems when they returned to Earth. Then NASA developed special exercises that create strain during space flights so astronauts' bones remain strong. Problem solved.

Most bone building takes place as the body reacts to changing or "dynamic" strain. Stand still for an hour and the hip and leg bones experience some strain. But it's static strain. It doesn't create much new bone. Walk for an hour and the strain is dynamic as we step, turn, crouch, climb, descend, and stretch to accommodate the terrain. That's why walking is a prime bone builder.

The bone-strengthening benefits of walking also make sense from an evolutionary perspective. We evolved from ancient apes that foraged widely for plant foods with occasional scavenging of meat. They walked all their lives. In other words, we evolved to walk long distances, dig for roots, and climb to pick fruit, with some running to hunt or escape threats.

Most studies of exercise and fracture risk have focused on walking or "leisure" activities, everything from gardening to Ping-Pong. But one Chinese study focused on the *types* of walking that are most fracture-preventive. The best were walking outdoors, walking up or down stairs or hills, and walking while carrying a load. This makes perfect sense. Walking outdoors over changing terrain is more dynamic than walking indoors on flat surfaces. And walking on stairs or hills or while carrying a load also increases dynamic strain.

Why Aren't Americans Active?

According to the CDC, healthy adults should be moderately physically active for at least 2.5 hours a week—30 minutes a day, 5 days a week. That's not much. Unfortunately, the latest CDC survey shows that fewer than half of Americans—just 48 percent—are this active.

Why are Americans so sedentary? Many reasons:

- **Less physical labor.** In 1950, 30 percent of American workers had jobs that required significant physical labor, while only 25 percent worked in offices. Today only 20 percent of the workforce has physically demanding jobs, and more than 40 percent work in offices.

- **More women working.** Until the 1960s, the most common occupation for women was homemaking and child rearing. Shopping, cleaning, washing, gardening, cooking from scratch, lifting and shepherding children, and other household chores involve considerable walking and lifting. Today many more women work outside the home in sedentary jobs. Most still do housework, but typically less than homemakers of previous generations. Others hire housecleaners, nannies, gardeners, and other helpers and do less of this physical work.

- **Longer commutes.** In 1950, only about half of Americans commuted to work by car. Today the figure is 80 percent. And commutes are longer than they were a generation ago. The result: more time spent sitting in cars and less time available to be active.

- **The growth of suburbs.** People who live in cities and in rural communities walk a good deal. Suburbs were created around the automobile. In many suburbs, residents must drive to accomplish anything. In 1950, 25 percent of Americans lived in suburbs. Today the figure is more than 50 percent as people move toward urban centers from rural areas and out of downtown in search of safer neighborhoods and a better life. The result: less walking.

- **Screen time.** Screens include TVs and computers. In 1960, the typical household spent less than four hours a day watching TV (total TV time by all family members). Today, the figure is eight hours—with plenty more time spent using computers.

- **Obesity.** All of the preceding factors conspire to add pounds to our bodies. As we gain weight, we have to expend more energy to move those extra pounds. Exercise becomes more difficult and tiring. The result: as body weight increases, activity tends to fall.

- **Finally, the aerobics error.** Many Americans believe that to improve health exercise must be aerobic, strenuous enough to raise the heart rate considerably. Wrong. Aerobic exercise is too strenuous for most people. They just don't enjoy it—hence all the home exercise machines that gather dust. Aerobic exercise also raises risk of injury.

Aerobic conditioning is necessary *only* if you're determined to excel at highly competitive sports (high school, college, Olympic, professional). If you're not a competitive athlete, if your exercise goal is health not trophies, then nonaerobic exercise is sufficient—assuming you do it *regularly*, ideally daily for at least half an hour. Nonaerobic exercise strengthens bone, improves sleep, controls weight, elevates mood (less anxiety and depression), enhances sex, and reduces risk of obesity, diabetes, high cholesterol, high blood pressure, heart disease, Alzheimer's, and many cancers.

The term "aerobic" was coined by Dallas physician Kenneth Cooper, M.D. In 1968, he published *Aerobics*, a bestseller that touted strenuous exercise just as Americans were waking up to the health benefits of fitness. Cooper had a military background. His research showed that for combat, or for intensely competitive athletics, heart-pounding aerobic conditioning provides a competitive advantage. Unfortunately, this observation was quickly corrupted into the notion that to provide any benefit, exercise *must be* aerobic.

Wrong—and ironically, this was proven by researchers at Cooper's own Cooper Institute for Aerobics Research in Dallas. Cooper scientists put 102 women on one of four exercise regimens: sedentary controls (no exercise), leisurely strolling (not aerobic, no sweating), brisk walking (not aerobic but working up a sweat after about twenty minutes), or racewalking (aerobic). The exercising groups all walked three miles five days a week for six months. Before-and-after tests charted changes in their health and fitness.

The aerobic racewalkers were the only group to improve their aerobic fitness. But the nonaerobic brisk walkers gained *the same health benefits*: lower cholesterol and lower blood pressure—and, compared with the racewalkers, they lost *more* weight.

Since then, many studies have shown that regular, nonaerobic exercise provides all the health benefits of strenuous aerobic workouts. (Aerobic fitness is *not* a health benefit. It provides a competitive edge.) In addition, walking, gardening, dancing, yoga, etc., offer two major advantages over aerobics: they are less strenuous, so people are more likely to stick with them, and nonaerobic exercise is less likely to cause injury so people *can* stick with it.

"We made a mistake telling everyone they had to engage in strenuous aerobic workouts at least three times a week to obtain health benefits from exercise," says Steven Blair, Ph.D., former director of epidemiology at the Cooper Institute. "Regular, moderate exercise is enough."

"The fitness gurus used to insist that we had to punish ourselves with strenuous aerobics for at least thirty minutes three times a week to become fit and healthy," says Bryant Stamford, Ph.D., director of the Health Promotion Center at the University of Louisville School of Medicine in Kentucky. "But major health benefits come from exercise so modest that it doesn't even feel like a 'workout.' "

The nation's health and fitness experts officially embraced moderate—that is, nonaerobic—exercise as the path to better health in 1995, when the CDC and the American College of Sports Medicine issued a joint report saying "If sedentary Americans adopted a more active lifestyle, there would be enormous benefits to individual well-being and the public health. An active lifestyle *does not require vigorous exercise.* Small lifestyle changes that increase daily activity are sufficient."

Five to Ten Thousand Steps

With walking, there's nothing to learn. You're already good at it. You don't have to join a gym. There's no clothing or equipment to buy. And you can carry on a conversation while walking, so it's sociable, a great way to spend time with friends. Just put one foot in front of the other and repeat.

The key to walking for stronger bones—and better health—is *regularity.* A half hour every day is preferable to one four-hour hike a week. To become a regular walker:

- Start smart. If you haven't been active in a while, see the section "If You're Just Getting Off the Couch."
- Make walking dates with your spouse, friends, parents, or kids.
- Commit to walking at the same time every day—before work or school, at lunch, after work, after dinner.
- Park a block or two farther away from your destination and walk a little more.
- If you're early for an appointment, don't sit in your car. Walk around the block.
- Invest in a treadmill. Place it in front of your TV. Whenever you watch TV, use it.
- Walk your dog. If you don't have a dog, but like dogs, consider getting one. Or walk a friend's dog.
- Look for opportunities to walk. Instead of yelling upstairs that dinner's ready, climb the stairs. Instead of using e-mail or the phone or intercom, walk to the person.
- When you're on the phone, pace back and forth.
- Take the stairs instead of the elevator or escalator. Start by walking *down.* That's easier than climbing stairs. Over time, as you become more conditioned, begin walking up. If you live or work on a high floor, begin by walking part of the way and take the elevator the rest of the way. Over time, walk up more flights.
- If you shop with friends, and they use the escalator, take the stairs and invite them to join you.
- Buy a pedometer. These little battery-powered devices contain computer chips that sense impact. They count your steps.

Health authorities recommend five to ten thousand steps a day, the equivalent of about two to four miles.

Pedometers encourage walking. If your daily goal is 5,000 steps, and you see you're at 4,639, you're likely to think, I'm so close. If I walk just a little more, I can get up to 5,000.

They allow easy charting of progress. Some models have thirty-day memories. But if your step-counter does not offer this feature, it's easy to jot down the date and how many steps you walked. As you continue walking, you gain fitness, so walking becomes easier. Your step total is likely to increase. You feel like you've accomplished something. You have.

Pedometers bring surprises. People who are not athletic sometimes assume they get *no* exercise. A pedometer can show that you're more active than you think. Keep one with you all day—clip it to clothing. That way you count every step everywhere you go. You'll be surprised by how many steps you take—and how many more you want to take once you can count them easily.

They're cheap. On the Internet, step-counting pedometers are available for $20 to $40.

Reduce Fractures by Preventing Falls

Osteoporotic fractures rarely occur spontaneously. A Johns Hopkins analysis of 169 people hospitalized with hip fractures shows that only two (1.2 percent) occurred for no apparent reason. An estimated 80 percent of osteoporotic fractures result from falls. (Most of the rest are caused by auto accidents.) Exercise improves limb strength, balance, and coordination at any age. Even for those who have been largely sedentary their entire lives, exercise reduces risk of falls—and the fractures they often cause.

We found seventeen studies dealing with falls and fractures:

- Fifteen (88 percent) show that exercise reduces risk of falling.
- One (6 percent) shows that exercise reduces falls—but the results were not statistically significant.

- One (6 percent) shows that exercise *increases* risk of falls. This study involved brisk walking—apparently too brisk for the older women involved.

The evidence is overwhelming that exercise reduces falls. It becomes even stronger when we look more closely at these studies. Several tested exercise-based fall-reduction programs. German researchers enrolled twenty-four older women in a three-month walking program. Afterward, the women were encouraged to continue walking on their own. After one year, compared with nonwalking controls, the walking women suffered an astonishing *89 percent fewer falls.* Other trials have not produced such dramatic results. But most studies show that regular walking reduces fall risk 40 to 60 percent—major decreases.

In addition to walking and other moderate exercise, improving balance helps prevent falls. Some activities that help improve balance include yoga, tai chi, and dance. Or practice this home balance-training program:

- Stand near a table or counter in case you need to steady yourself.
- Stand straight. Extend your arms at shoulder height, forming a T.
- With eyes open, lift one leg, bending your knee in front of you. Work up to holding this pose for a slow count of twenty.
- Repeat, balancing on the other leg.
- With eyes open, lift one leg off the floor and extend it behind you. Work up to holding this pose for a slow count of twenty.
- Repeat both lifts with eyes open and arms folded across your chest.
- Repeat all of these steps with eyes closed.

Fall-Proofing Your Home

You've heard of childproofing—simple adjustments around the house that keep toddlers from getting hurt. People at risk for osteoporotic fractures should fall-proof their homes:

- Eliminate area rugs, runners, and mats. They're tripping hazards. Install wall-to-wall carpet.
- Don't wax floors. It makes them slippery.
- Don't run electrical cords across traffic paths.
- Add more night-lights.
- If you don't have grab-bar railings on stairs, tubs, and showers, install them.
- If stairs need repair, fix them.
- Use a nonslip mat in your tub/shower.
- Eliminate clutter on floors.
- Invest in a step stool with a handrail.
- Repair damaged sidewalks.
- Keep steps, sidewalks, and driveways clear of snow and ice. If you can't manage this, hire someone who can.

If You're Just Getting Off the Couch

Even if you haven't exercised in years, you can start today and immediately begin to gain health benefits, including less risk of osteoporosis. If you have a chronic condition (diabetes, high blood pressure, heart disease), it's best to consult your doctor before starting an exercise program.

- **Wear comfortable clothes and shoes.** Clothing should feel loose enough to allow for easy movement. Shoes should fit well and not chafe.

- **Don't overdo it.** Walking for health should be enjoyable, not exhausting. Walk at a pace that feels comfortable. Don't dawdle, but don't become winded. You should be able to talk comfortably while walking. If you find yourself gasping for breath as you talk, you're walking too briskly.

- **If you carry anything, use a backpack.** Carrying things in hand is tiring and interferes with the natural rhythm of walking. A backpack allows your arms to swing freely, which helps prevent fatigue.

Risk Factors for Falling

In addition to lack of exercise, risk factors for falls include:

- **Alcohol.** Even one drink impairs balance. A Finnish study of 222 people with hip fractures shows that at hospitalization almost one person in five—19 percent of the men and 16 percent of the women—had alcohol in their bloodstreams.
- **High heels.** They interfere with balance. Whenever possible, women should wear flats.
- **Poor eyesight.** If you can't see hazards, you might trip over them and fall. Have your vision checked regularly and corrected appropriately.
- **Drowsiness.** Sleepiness interferes with awareness of tripping hazards. Most adults need seven to nine hours of sleep a night to avoid daytime drowsiness.
- **Knee pain.** Osteoarthritis of the knee is common among older people and makes them less sure on their feet. Regular, moderate exercise helps control osteoarthritis pain. Beyond that, over-the-counter pain relievers help. Or see your physician.
- **Narcotics, tranquilizers, and sedatives.** These drugs increase risk of falls. Exercise has a tranquilizing effect that relieves stress and improves sleep. If you exercise daily, you may not need these drugs.
- **Frailty.** It's associated with poor fitness, postural sway, and poor vision.

- **Focus on how you feel afterward.** Don't expect euphoria. Instead, enjoy the strange combination of weariness, invigoration, and mood elevation that exercise produces. Assuming you didn't overdo it, fatigue passes quickly, but feelings of invigoration and emotional uplift last longer. As you continue walking, your physical condition improves. You'll feel less fatigue and more invigoration and mood elevation.

- **Warm up beforehand.** Walking slowly for the first five minutes is usually sufficient.

- **Progress slowly.** The body needs time to adjust to increased physical activity. If you don't allow sufficient adjustment time, you won't have fun and you risk injury. Start by walking every third day for four weeks. Then walk every other day for a month. Then walk three days in a row and take a day off; then walk four or five days in a row with one day off. Finally, walk every day.

- **Chart your progress.** A pedometer helps. Charting progress reminds you how far you've come and provides a sense of accomplishment that helps walking become a permanent part of your life.

- **Set modest goals and reward yourself.** Instead of a banana split, reward yourself with walking-oriented treats: a new pair of walking shoes, some new socks, or a weekend at a country inn near inviting hiking trails.

- **Refine your technique.** Don't march. Instead, flow forward. Roll your foot from heel to toe. When walking uphill, slow down, lean forward, and put more energy into your arm swing. When walking downhill, maintain a comfortable speed, take shorter steps, and don't slap your feet down. That's hard on the ankles, knees, and hips. Instead, plant your feet gently.

- **Skip your coffee break.** A jolt of caffeine can boost productivity. But so can a quick ten-minute walk. If you're still dragging at the end of a walk break, have that cup of coffee. But chances are you won't need it.

Weight and Fractures: Obesity Is Bad for Health, but It Reduces Fracture Risk

Obesity shortens life expectancy because it increases risk of diabetes, high cholesterol, high blood pressure, heart disease, stroke, and many cancers. But according to many studies, fractures are much more likely in those who are underweight (especially frail) than overweight. Extra weight means more bone strain during weight-bearing exercise and, as a result, more new bone and stronger bones.

In some ways this is counterintuitive. People who are obese may eat a diet high in animal foods, fast food, and junk food and low in fruits and vegetables. That diet increases fracture risk. People who are obese also tend to be sedentary. Lack of exercise increases fracture risk. Finally, people who are obese often develop type 2 diabetes, a major risk factor for fractures (Chapter 14).

Nonetheless, being overweight or obese reduces fracture risk. Why? Because despite all the reasons why obesity should increase fracture risk, extra weight increases bone strain and bone formation. Decreased fracture risk is no reason to become overweight. But it shows how important weight-bearing exercise is to bone strength and fracture prevention.

Exercise Is Crucial to Children's Bone Development

Among the sixty-eight trials that correlate exercise and fracture risk, nine focus specifically on young people:

- Seven studies (78 percent) show that exercise while young reduces fracture risk from youth to old age.
- One (11 percent) shows that childhood exercise has no effect on fracture risk at any age.
- One (11 percent) shows that exercise during youth *increases* fracture risk.

Let's take a closer look at the one study showing that youthful exercise increases fracture risk. Harvard researchers analyzed diet, lifestyle, and fractures among 5,461 girls aged eleven to seventeen. Compared with those who exercised for less than thirty minutes a day, girls who exercised for more than two hours a day had almost double the fracture risk. But the exercising girls did not engage in moderate exercise that reduces risk of fractures. They participated in high-impact sports—mostly running, cheerleading, and gymnastics. High-impact means greater fracture risk. And these are sports where athletes may limit food intake to meet specific body weight or size ideals for their sport. Even with the high-impact study in the analysis, a compelling 78 percent of trials support regular exercise from cradle to grave as crucial to bone strength throughout life. Eliminating this study, seven of eight trials (88 percent) show that exercise while young reduces fracture risk throughout life.

Two of these studies calculated numerical decreases in fracture risk:

- Columbia University researchers asked 329 elderly women—161 with hip factures and 168 matched controls—how active they were as teens. Compared with the women who were least active when young, the most active were 76 percent less likely to suffer a hip fracture. Of course, this study suffers from the problem inherent in retrospective studies, inaccurate recall. Even allowing for this, the effect size is enormous. Compared with the women who recalled little exercise as teens, those who were active had only *one-quarter* of the fracture risk.
- Researchers at the University of Toronto conducted a similar study involving 381 women with hip fractures and 1,138 matched controls. Compared with the least active, women who were most active were 46 percent less likely to suffer hip fracture.

Overall, it looks like regular moderate exercise during youth reduces the risk of osteoporotic hip fracture by 40 to 60 percent.

The best the conventional wisdom has to offer—calcium plus vitamin D—reduces risk about 17 percent. Even without low-acid eating, compared with calcium and vitamin D, exercise provides about *three times the benefit.*

Bottom line: parents should encourage kids to engage in as much physically active play as possible.

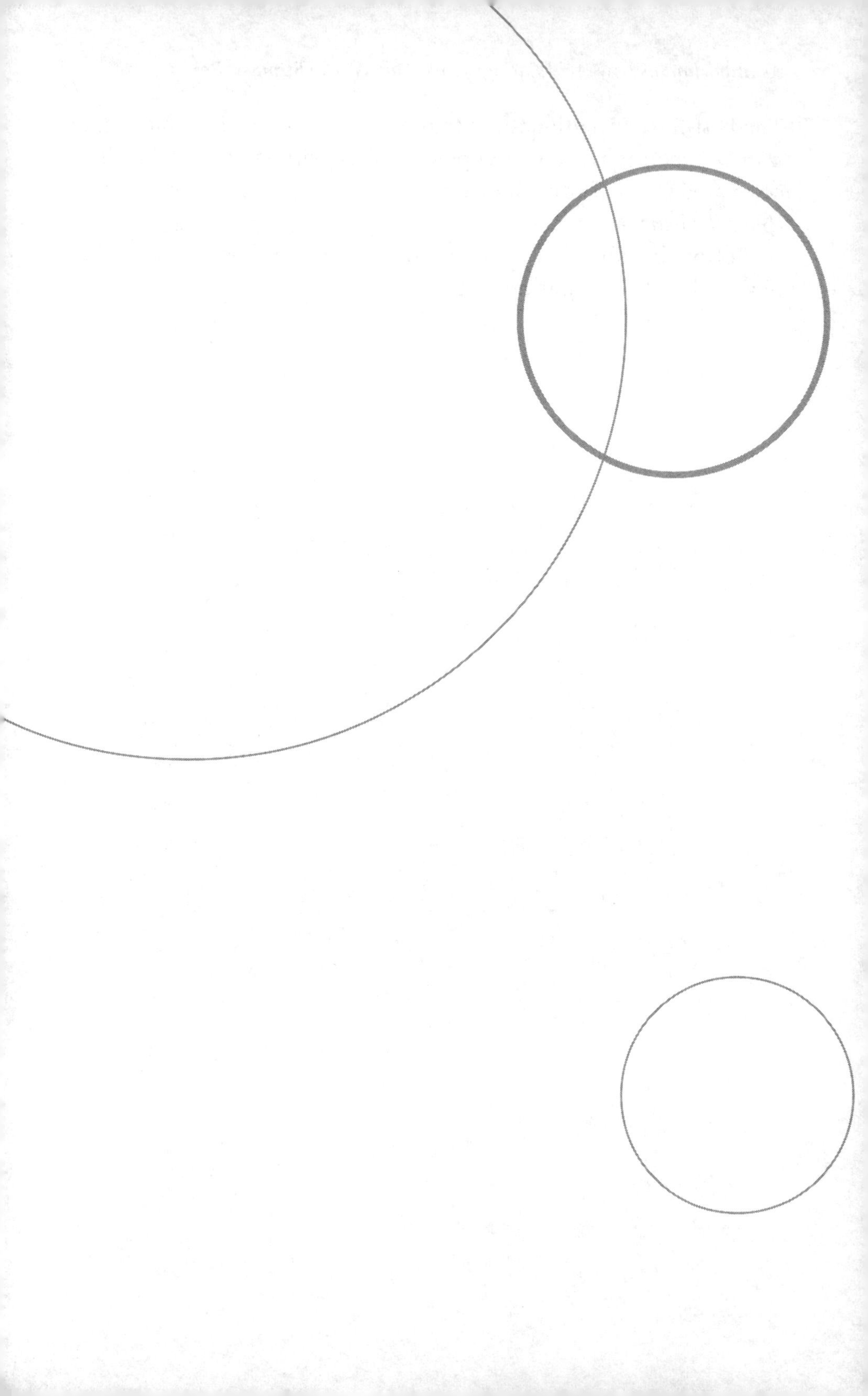

PART 3

Other Risk Factors for Osteoporosis and What You Can Do About Them

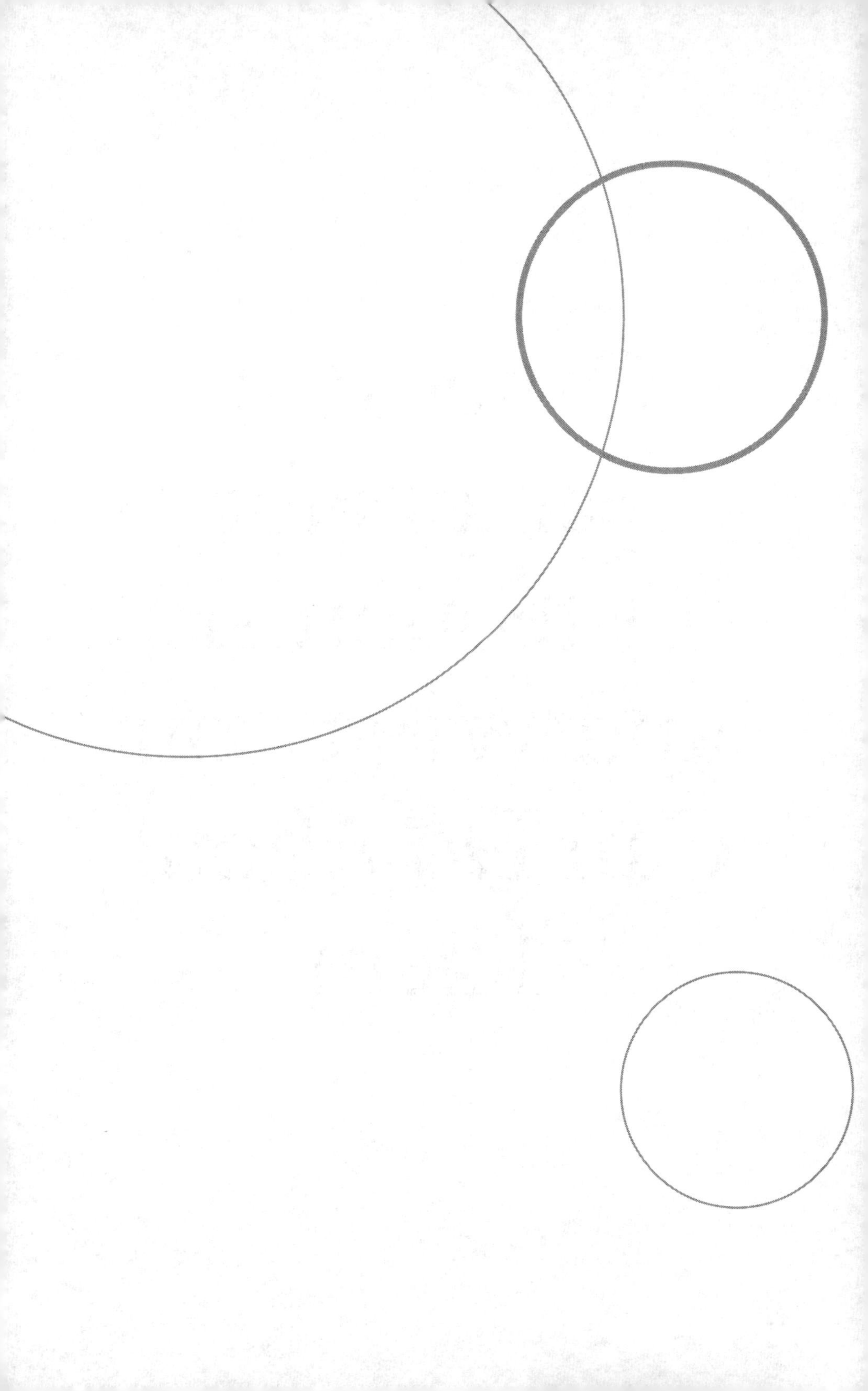

Diabetes, Frailty, and Fractures

SEVERAL CHRONIC DISEASES are associated with bone loss and fractures, among them epilepsy, kidney failure, HIV/AIDS, rheumatoid arthritis, and chronic obstructive pulmonary disease (COPD). In some cases the disease itself leads to fractures. During seizures, people may fall and break bones. In others the treatment increases fracture risk. People with COPD may take steroids, which harm bone. (See Chapter 15.) But fractures are most strongly associated with two chronic conditions—diabetes and frailty.

Diabetes Is a Major Risk Factor for Fractures

More than two thousand years ago the ancients noticed that some people produced copious amounts of strangely sweet-smelling urine. They named the condition *diabetes mellitus*, from the Greek for "fountain" and the Latin for "honey." Doctors continue to call this condition *diabetes mellitus* or *DM*, but in common parlance, it's just *diabetes*.

Diabetes develops when the body stops producing the pancreatic hormone insulin or can't use the insulin the pancreas makes.

Without insulin, the body's major fuel, blood sugar (glucose), cannot enter the cells. Sugar builds up in the bloodstream and eventually turns up in urine, making it sweet.

If someone spills Coca-Cola in a movie theater, the floor gets sticky. Something similar happens in the blood vessels when diabetes raises blood sugar. Sticky, sugary blood triggers biochemical changes that injure the blood vessels. Over time these injuries cause the many complications of the disease.

There are two types of diabetes. In type 1, the body can't make insulin. Everyone with type 1 diabetes must inject it daily. But type 1 diabetes accounts for only 5 percent of the disease. Ninety-five percent of people with diabetes have type 2. The pancreas continues to produce insulin, but the body's cells become "insulin resistant" and can't use it.

What causes insulin resistance? Biochemical changes associated with the risk factors for obesity—little or no exercise and a diet low in fruits and vegetables and high in sugar, fat, and animal foods. Not all people with type 2 diabetes are overweight or obese, but the large majority are. If you are wondering if you are overweight or at risk for diabetes, ask your doctor.

We found twenty-two studies of fracture risk in people with type 2 diabetes:

- Twenty (91 percent) show that it's a strong risk factor for fractures.
- Two studies (9 percent) show that type 2 diabetes has no effect on fracture risk.

The evidence is very compelling that type 2 diabetes makes fracture risk soar:

- Norwegian researchers followed 27,159 residents of Tromso, Norway, for six years. Compared with healthy people, those with type 2 diabetes had *nine times* the fracture risk.

- Other Norwegian scientists tracked diabetes and hip fractures in 52,313 older adults for thirteen years. Compared with nondiabetics, diabetes raised fracture risk *seven times.*
- Swedish scientists followed 33,346 adults starting at age forty-four. After sixteen years, compared with those who did not have diabetes, those with type 2 suffered almost *four times* as many hip fractures.
- For twenty-two years Harvard researchers followed 109,983 women nurses, some of whom had type 2 diabetes. Compared with healthy nurses, those who had type 2 suffered twice as many fractures.

The reasons for the link between osteoporotic fractures and type 2 diabetes remain unclear. But people with type 2 are often overweight, suggesting a diet high in animal foods. In addition, compared with healthy people, people with diabetes tend to be less physically active, have generally poorer balance and coordination, are often less steady on their feet, and fall more. Finally, diabetes damages most body systems. It makes sense that it would damage bone. Whatever the reasons, the evidence is overwhelming that type 2 diabetes substantially increases fracture risk.

Type 2 diabetes is increasingly prevalent. An estimated 20 million Americans have it.

Meanwhile, type 2 diabetes can be reversed to the point where drugs and insulin are no longer necessary. How? By eating a low-fat, low-acid diet and engaging in regular, moderate exercise. In fact, Dr. Neal Barnard and colleagues helped people with type 2 diabetes move to a vegan diet. When they did, they were able to improve, and in some cases reverse, their diabetes without counting calories or adding exercise to their daily routine. Many people with type 2 diabetes revert to normal blood sugar and eliminate insulin resistance if they lose 10 to 20 percent of their weight—twenty to forty pounds for a person weighing 200. In other words, the program we recommend to prevent osteoporosis also prevents—and reverses—type 2 diabetes and the increased risk of fractures associated with it.

Thinness, Frailty, and Fractures

Compared with those who maintain recommended weight, people who weigh less have lower bone mineral density and greater risk of fractures. In addition, significant weight loss after age sixty-five is a major risk factor for fractures.

We found 51 studies that correlated low body mass index with risk of osteoporotic fractures:

- Forty-two trials (82 percent) show that weighing less than health authorities recommend increases fracture risk.
- Two (4 percent) are inconclusive.
- Five (10 percent) show that low weight has no effect on fracture risk.
- And two (4 percent) show that being thinner than recommended reduces fracture risk.

This is strong evidence that being unusually thin boosts fracture risk. Why? This is the flip side of obesity's being somewhat protective against fractures. (See Chapter 13.) Being underweight, thin, slight, or petite means that during weight-bearing activity the bones support less weight and experience less strain, hence less bone building. If you're thin, in addition to low-acid eating, consider walking wearing a backpack containing weight (groceries, water bottles, etc.) to increase bone strain and bone formation.

In people over sixty-five, significant weight loss is a key sign of frailty. Other frailty-related changes include poor balance and loss of muscle strength, coordination, and appetite, all of which increase risk of falling and fractures. Frailty is very common among nursing home residents, the group with a very high risk of fracture.

Risk Factors for Fractures? Salt, Caffeine, Alcohol, Smoking, Depression, and Several Prescription Drugs

OVER THE PAST thirty years, dozens of studies have accused salt, caffeine, alcohol, smoking, and some prescription drugs of increasing osteoporotic fracture risk. Some of these do, indeed, boost fracture risk. Others don't. And moderate amounts of one might even help *prevent* fractures.

Halt the Salt?

A high-salt diet is bad for health. Salt (sodium chloride) raises blood pressure and is a risk factor for heart disease and especially for stroke.

Several studies show that as dietary salt increases, so does calcium in urine. This finding raises the possibility that a high-salt diet might be a risk factor for osteoporosis.

Only a few studies have investigated this—no fracture trials, just studies of salt's effects on bone mineral density.

We found six trials:

- Three (50 percent) show that a high-salt diet reduces BMD.
- Three (50 percent) show a high-salt diet has no effect on BMD.

Neither group of studies appears notably more credible than the other. So, is salt a risk factor for osteoporosis?

Researchers doubt it. British scientists conclude: "The limited studies to date indicate that increased sodium intake does not exert a consistent effect on biomarkers of bone health. We conclude that increased salt intake is not an important risk factor for osteoporosis."

Croatian researchers concur: "Sodium [salt] effects on bone are inconsistent. There is no evidence that increased salt intake is a risk factor for osteoporosis."

Most salt in the American diet comes not from the saltshaker but from snack and junk foods (potato chips, corn chips, etc.), processed foods (TV dinners, convenience foods, canned soups, soy sauce, ketchup), and fast foods (especially french fries). Fruits and vegetables are very low in salt. Indeed, one study shows that for those who consume a great deal of salt, a diet high in fruits and vegetables substantially lowers calcium excreted in urine.

For prevention of high blood pressure, heart disease, and stroke, limit your salt intake. The best way to do this is to eat a diet based on fruits and vegetables, the low-acid diet we recommend. Whether or not salt turns out to be a significant risk factor for fractures, the low-acid diet that prevents osteoporosis is very low in salt.

Caffeine: What the Buzz Does

Caffeine has many effects on health, some harmful, some beneficial, some neutral. Downsides include insomnia, jitters, irritability, and increased risk of migraines and, in women, infertility and miscarriage. Caffeine benefits include increased strength, stamina, and mental acuity and reduced risk of gallstones, Parkinson's disease, and nonmigraine headaches.

Caffeine, specifically coffee, has also been accused of increasing risk of heart disease, cancer, diabetes, high blood pressure, and premenstrual syndrome. But the weight of the evidence shows that moderate caffeine consumption—up to two cups a day of brewed coffee or up to four cups of tea—does not increase risk of these conditions.

What about osteoporosis? Several studies show that caffeine increases calcium excretion in urine, raising the possibility that it might increase fracture risk.

We found twenty-three trials of caffeine and fractures:

- Ten studies (43 percent) show that caffeine increases fracture risk.
- Four (17 percent) are inconclusive.
- Nine (39 percent) show that caffeine has no effect on fracture risk.

In terms of scientific credibility, four of the ten studies showing that caffeine boosts fractures are prospective—up to 34,703 participants followed for up to twelve years. Meanwhile, three of the studies showing no effect are also prospective—up to 91,465 participants followed for up to thirteen years.

The evidence tilts slightly toward caffeine as a risk factor for fractures. But it's far from compelling.

However, there may be a simple explanation for why the large, long-term prospective trials disagree. It looks as though there's a caffeine threshold for fracture risk. Having up to two cups of coffee a day (four cups a day of tea or cola) does not increase risk. But any more does. Most coffee drinkers consume only one to two cups a day, below the threshold for caffeine-related bone damage. If you limit coffee to two cups a day or less (four cups of tea), you probably don't have to worry about the caffeine contributing to fractures. But if you drink more, you might consider cutting down to protect your bones.

Speaking of caffeine, parents may want to discourage cola drinking in kids. Several studies show that caffeinated colas increase the risk of childhood fractures.

But among soft drinks, *only* caffeinated colas are associated with fractures. Carbonation, per se, does not appear to increase risk. One bit of osteoporosis lore holds that carbonated beverages dissolve bone. But the evidence shows that only colas have any association with fractures. Current evidence suggests that the problem is large amounts of caffeine, *not* carbonation.

Booze and Bones: Heavy Drinking Increases Fractures; A Little Alcohol May Prevent Them

There are many reasons why heavy drinking should raise risk of fractures. Alcohol:

- suppresses the activity of bone-building osteoblasts;
- impairs balance, increasing the risk of falls;
- is linked to poor nutrition—fewer fruits and vegetables;
- is associated with smoking (more on smoking later in this chapter); and
- irritates the stomach lining and is associated with use of antacids (see the end of this chapter).

We found thirty-seven studies of alcohol's effects on fracture risk:

- Fifteen (41 percent) show that alcohol increases risk of fractures.
- One (3 percent) is inconclusive.
- Eleven (30 percent) show that alcohol has no effect on fracture risk.
- Nine (24 percent) show that moderate alcohol consumption—one to two drinks a day—helps prevent fractures but that drinking any more increases risk.
- And one study (3 percent) shows that as alcohol use increases, fracture risk decreases.

The data lean toward alcohol as a fracture risk, but given all the reasons why this should be true, it's odd that the research is not more one-sided.

Among the large, long-duration prospective trials, six (60 percent) show that alcohol boosts fracture risk. Four (40 percent) show it doesn't. More studies show that alcohol increases fractures. They are also larger and longer. But not all that many more, and some of the studies showing no effect are quite large—51,529 people followed for six years. If alcohol really increases fracture risk, wouldn't such a large, extended study likely show it?

Then there's the issue of moderate alcohol consumption. Does it *really* reduce fracture risk? Based on current evidence, that's hard to say. If moderate alcohol consumption protects against fractures, the biochemical reason remains unclear. In addition, several of the studies linking alcohol to increased fracture risk show rising risk with *any* drinking, even the moderate drinking other studies call protective. This issue is far from settled.

Finally, alcohol-health considerations involve much more than just fracture risk. Very compelling evidence links moderate drinking—up to one drink a day for most women and up to two for most men—to reduced risk of heart disease. Meanwhile, strong evidence shows that even a few drinks a week increases risk of breast cancer. So when considering whether or not to drink, and if so, how much, women have a great deal to ponder.

Here's what we think: no one should abuse alcohol, which means no one should drink more than one or two drinks a day. If you drink moderately or only occasionally, ask your doctor about your risk for heart disease, breast cancer, and osteoporosis and then make the decision that feels right to you.

Bones Up in Smoke

Beyond vastly increasing the risk of lung cancer, heart disease, and several other serious conditions, smoking increases the risk of osteoporotic fractures. We found sixty-two studies:

- Forty-three (69 percent) show that smoking increases fracture risk.
- Four (6 percent) are inconclusive.
- Fifteen (24 percent) show that smoking has no effect on fracture risk.

More than two-thirds of studies link smoking to fractures. Even if smoking didn't cause a host of other life-threatening conditions, that would be pretty compelling evidence to quit.

Smoking loads the bloodstream with highly reactive oxygen ions that cause the cell damage, oxidative damage, that is at the root of all the havoc smoking wreaks.

Oxidative damage can be prevented with antioxidant nutrients, among them vitamins C and E. Several studies show that as dietary antioxidants increase, fracture risk decreases—even among smokers. This parallels findings on lung cancer. Smokers who consume the most antioxidants are to some extent protected. Antioxidant nutrients are found only in plant foods. Eating a plant-based, low-acid diet supplies plenty of them.

Antioxidant supplements are another option. But compared with studies of fruits and vegetables, the research in favor of supplements for prevention of heart disease, cancer, and fractures is considerably less compelling. For health, the best way to obtain all the antioxidant nutrients is to eat a low-acid diet.

For those who quit smoking, fracture risk remains high for about ten years and then returns to average.

Depression: In the Mood for Fractures

When people feel anxious, stressed, or depressed, they produce more of the hormone cortisol. Eventually it shows up in their urine. High levels of urinary cortisol are associated with decreased bone mineral density. Do anxiety, stress, and depression increase fracture risk?

Although no studies have investigated anxiety and stress as risk factors for fracture, eleven trials have focused on depression and fall/fracture risk in older adults. All eleven (100 percent) show that depressed mood—or taking antidepressant medication—increases the risk of both falls and fractures.

Some studies show that, compared with those who are not depressed, those who are suffer only slightly increased fall/fracture risk. Others show that depression increases fall/fracture risk by as much as five times. Overall, it looks like depression approximately doubles the risk of falls and fractures.

Depression is serious, the main risk factor for suicide. Anyone whose mood remains bleak for more than two weeks should consult a physician and psychotherapist.

Beyond medical treatment and psychotherapy, an effective mood elevator is exercise. Physical activity releases endorphins, the body's own antidepressant/feel-good compounds. Exercise also strengthens bone and prevents fractures. So those who feel depressed—from normal blues to clinical depression—can help their mood and their bones by walking or getting other exercise.

Rx for Fractures?

Finally, several prescription drugs increase fracture risk:

- **Valium, other tranquilizers, and sedatives.** Five studies link the use of these drugs to increased fracture risk. No studies show otherwise. It makes perfect sense that tranquilizers and sedatives would increase fracture risk. Like alcohol, these drugs make people less sure on their feet and more likely to fall.

- **Avandia, Actos.** These widely prescribed diabetes drugs suppress bone-forming osteoblasts. In a Swiss case-control study involving 4,748 adults, taking either of these drugs for a year more than doubled fracture risk.

- **Steroids.** These anti-inflammatory drugs (prednisone and others) are used widely to treat conditions like colitis and Crohn's disease. Steroids suppress osteoblasts. Long-term use is associated with fractures. We found eleven reports documenting this and none disputing it.

- **Seizure medication.** Anticonvulsant drugs are also strongly associated with fractures. We found five studies documenting this and none concluding otherwise.

- **Prilosec, Nexium, Prevacid, and other proton pump inhibitors (PPIs).** To date the research is scant—only two studies. But both show that these widely prescribed antacids/heartburn treatments increase fracture risk in older adults. PPIs reduce calcium absorption in the digestive tract. While two studies don't prove that PPIs increase fracture risk, no research shows otherwise. Fortunately, there are nondrug approaches to chronic heartburn, among them a dairy-free, plant-based diet and regular exercise. So in addition to reducing risk of fractures, our recommendations might also help people taking PPIs get off them.

Most of the drug studies deal with people over sixty-five, and often frail, very old nursing home residents. The risk to younger people is less clear.

Taking any of these drugs does not doom anyone to fractures. It simply increases risk. If you take any of these drugs, it would be prudent to embrace low-acid eating and daily weight-bearing exercise.

Should You Take Osteoporosis Drugs?

HERE'S WHAT YOU need to know about the drugs currently prescribed to reduce the risk of osteoporotic fractures:

- They work reasonably well, but they're no cure—not even close.
- The drug industry exaggerates their effectiveness, and at least some of the hyperbole rubs off on doctors, who then overestimate the drugs' effectiveness to the public.
- The drugs have been tested only against placebos or, in some cases, each other or calcium and vitamin D. They have never been tested against low-acid eating and daily walking. As a result, we have no way of knowing how they stack up against diet and lifestyle approaches. However, based on the evidence presented in Chapters 7 and 13, it appears that low-acid eating and daily walking reduce fracture risk as effectively—or better—though the drugs work faster.
- The drugs often cause side effects that range from annoying to, rarely, life-threatening. The only side effects of low-acid eating and regular, moderate exercise are beneficial—substantially

lower risk of heart disease, stroke, cancer, obesity, diabetes, high blood pressure, and Alzheimer's disease.

- Finally, a safe, very cheap generic drug that's been around for decades strengthens bone almost as much as the osteoporosis drugs—but doctors don't prescribe it.

We have nothing against drugs for those who truly need them, particularly people who have suffered osteoporotic fractures, those who are frail and/or at high risk of fracture, and/or those who take any of the drugs that substantially raise fracture risk, notably steroids. But for everyone else, low-acid eating and daily walking make much more sense. They're as effective as, or more effective than, the drugs. They're also cheaper, safer, and better for overall heath.

Hormone Replacement Therapy: A Cautionary Tale

Before we delve into the osteoporosis drugs, it's instructive to discuss their most widely prescribed predecessor, postmenopausal hormone replacement therapy (HRT)—estrogen alone or estrogen plus progestin/progesterone. For years public health officials and osteoporosis experts touted HRT as the answer to bone loss and fractures—until it turned out that its cost (deaths from heart attack, stroke, and breast cancer) outweighed its benefits (fewer fractures and less colon cancer).

HRT is not the only drug to experience a meteoric rise and fall. Many drugs have been approved by the Food and Drug Administration and touted by researchers, only to have subsequent studies show more harm than good. To be fair, the benefits of the drugs currently prescribed to prevent and treat osteoporotic fractures appear to outweigh their risks. But nasty surprises may still lurk down the road.

The HRT story begins in 1966 when *Feminine Forever* by Robert Wilson, M.D., became a bestseller. Wilson argued that, like people with diabetes who replace insulin, older women should replace estrogen, which declines after menopause. He said HRT, specifically the drug Premarin, eliminated hot flashes and made women "more attractive and much more pleasant to live with." Wilson presented himself as an independent researcher. But according to the *New York Times*, the maker of Premarin, Wyeth-Ayerst, subsidized him while writing the book and financed his promotional efforts.

Millions of women took Premarin. It did, indeed, eliminate hot flashes. But this common discomfort of menopause can also be minimized with a variety of nondrug approaches, among them a low-fat (10 to 15 percent of calories) vegetarian diet, regular exercise, the medicinal herb black cohosh (Remifemin), and, according to some reports, soy foods.

As HRT became popular, laboratory research showed that it suppressed osteoclasts. This raised the possibility that it might reduce fractures. Indeed, from the 1970s into the 1990s, observational studies showed that HRT cut osteoporotic fractures roughly 40 percent. Other studies showed that HRT reduced risk of heart disease, stroke, colon cancer, and Alzheimer's disease. Unfortunately, HRT also increased risk of breast, ovarian, and uterine (endometrial) cancers.

But the nation's health experts insisted that for most women HRT's benefits outweighed its risks. During the 1990s about 35 percent of American women died from heart disease, stroke, and colon cancer. Meanwhile, women's risk of dying from breast, ovarian, and endometrial cancers was less than 10 percent. Women with personal or family histories of these cancers were advised to avoid HRT. But leading medical organizations—including the American College of Physicians, the American College of Family Medicine, and the U.S. Preventive Services Task Force—encouraged most other women to take hormones. At the height of HRT's popularity, American doctors wrote eighty million prescriptions a year.

But during the 1980s researchers began raising questions about HRT. Did it really decrease the risk of heart attack and stroke? The studies showed these results. But the studies were observational. They simply looked at what happened over time to large groups of women who either took HRT or didn't. And compared with women who did not take HRT, hormone users were, on average, better educated, weighed less, exercised more, and had lower cholesterol and blood pressure. In other words, even *without* HRT, hormone users would be expected to have lower rates of heart disease and stroke. Several moderate-sized prospective trials showed no HRT-related decreases in heart attack and stroke. Ominously, some showed *increased* risk.

To determine the effects of HRT once and for all, in 1991 the National Institutes of Health launched the Women's Health Initiative, a prospective trial involving more than 90,000 U.S. women, 16,608 of whom were postmenopausal and took either HRT or a placebo. The study was supposed to last eight years. But in 2002, after just five years, it was terminated. A preliminary analysis showed that, as expected, the group taking HRT suffered less colon cancer and 40 percent fewer hip fractures. But HRT *increased* the risk of heart disease, stroke, and pulmonary embolisms (potentially fatal blood clots in the lungs). Bottom line: HRT did more harm than good.

Subsequently, other large prospective trials confirmed HRT as a risk factor for heart disease, stroke, and pulmonary embolism. HRT use plummeted.

Most recently, University of North Carolina researchers reported that even several years after terminating HRT, women who took it remain at increased risk of heart disease, stroke, pulmonary embolism, breast cancer, and death from all causes.

Today, Premarin is rarely prescribed. Women debilitated by severe hot flashes or other menopausal discomforts are usually prescribed a skin patch that delivers a much lower dose of estrogen, a dose not associated with the problems caused by high-dose, oral HRT.

How Effective Are Osteoporosis Drugs Really?

Page through the medical journals that publish osteoporosis research, or the medical magazines sent to the doctors who treat it, and you see big, splashy advertisements for osteoporosis drugs. Invariably, they contain large, colorful bar graphs showing that the drugs produce huge reductions in fractures. Headlines proclaim: 65 percent fewer fractures! That sounds pretty impressive. But is it true?

Yes and no.

The most widely prescribed osteoporosis drug is Fosamax (alendronate). We found nine meta-analyses that pooled the results of up to eleven trials involving as many as 12,068 people who took it for one to four years. At first glance, Fosamax appears to reduce fracture risk 45 to 65 percent, half to two-thirds.

But on closer examination these reductions relate to fractures of the *vertebrae*, the bones that surround the spine. Of the annual 1.5 million osteoporotic fractures in the United States, vertebral, or compression, fractures account for 700,000 of them, or 47 percent. Reducing risk of vertebral fractures by half to two-thirds is great news for elderly people who have already suffered one and for those with low bone mineral density who want to avoid spending their final years stooped over or with back deformities (so-called *dowager's hump*) or suffering the pain and disability that vertebral fractures often cause.

But while vertebral fractures account for almost half of osteoporotic fractures, they account for a considerably smaller proportion of the $18 billion the United States spends on osteoporosis every year. The costliest fractures by far are hip fractures. Vertebral fractures may or may not send people to hospitals. Hip fractures always do. Vertebral fractures by themselves rarely send people into nursing homes. Hip fractures often do. Vertebral fractures are not a significant predictor of terminal decline. Hip fractures are.

Two of the Fosamax meta-analyses broke out hip fractures separately and found risk reductions of around 45 percent. Now, 45 percent fewer hip fractures is nothing to sneeze at. But these figures are notably lower than the 65 percent reductions trumpeted in Fosamax advertising.

Another problem with drug industry effectiveness figures: In clinical trials, some people don't take the medication as directed. But most do. In research studies, rates of what doctors call *drug compliance* are high. Participants know they're involved in a clinical trial.

They agree to take the drug (or placebo) as directed. Then periodically (or often) the researchers remind them.

In real life, compliance rates are lower, often much lower. Some people are forgetful. Many dislike taking medicine. The drugs have side effects. And the Fosamax family of drugs must be taken first thing in the morning on an empty stomach, requiring users to avoid eating anything for thirty minutes, which can be a hassle. As a result, clinical trials overestimate the drugs' actual effectiveness in the real world. Italian researchers gave Fosamax to 880 women with osteoporosis and then, after at least one year, compared their fracture rates with rates in the clinical trials that got these drugs approved. The fracture rate in this real-world study was "considerably higher than that observed in clinical trials."

In medical journal reports such as the meta-analyses we mention, the authors are usually careful to distinguish between the drugs' effectiveness against vertebral and nonvertebral fractures. But few doctors spend major blocks of time delving deeply into the medical literature. They're too busy treating patients. They get their drug-effectiveness information from a variety of sources. But a big one is the drug companies—salespeople, direct-to-doctor advertising, advertising in medical journals and trade publications, and lavish displays at medical meetings and continuing medical education seminars (often sponsored by the drug industry).

It's certainly possible to ignore advertising. But there's a reason the drug industry spends hundreds of millions of dollars a year to influence doctors' prescribing habits. It works. When doctors see ad after ad in journal after journal claiming 65 percent fewer fractures, they might forget that, for the fractures that matter most, hip fractures, the figure is at best 45 percent and is actually considerably lower because of noncompliance. When doctors get the wrong impression, so does the public.

Finally, even if everyone took Fosamax precisely as directed, it would reduce hip fractures by about half. But that's no better than the benefits produced by low-acid eating and daily walking—and it's *less* than many diet/exercise studies show. The diet-and-lifestyle approach is also cheaper and safer, and all the side effects are beneficial.

The Other Bisphosphonates

Fosamax is just one of the bisphosphonates, a group of medications that are currently the drugs of choice for treating low bone mineral density. They are the safest, most thoroughly researched osteoporosis medications, and the most widely prescribed, with sales of more than $4 billion a year in the United States alone. Besides Fosamax (alendronate), they include Actonel (risedronate), Didronel (etidronate), Boniva (ibandronate), Zometa or Reclast (zoledronic acid), and Aredia (pamidronate). You've already read about Fosamax; research we found on the other bisphosphonates follows.

- **Actonel (risedronate).** We found six meta-analyses of up to eleven trials that followed as many as 14,049 people for up to three years. Actonel reduces the risk of vertebral fractures 37 percent. But it's much less effective against hip fracture, just 22 percent—substantially less effective than low-acid eating and daily walking.

- **Didronel (etidronate).** Four meta-analyses examined up to 13 trials lasting at least a year and involving up to 1,248 people. Didronel reduces vertebral fractures 46 percent but has *no effect* on hip, arm, and wrist fractures.

- **Boniva (ibandronate).** Three meta-analyses looked at up to thirteen studies involving as many as 8,710 people tracked for up to three years. Boniva reduces the risk of vertebral fractures by about one-third. One meta-analysis shows the drug cuts risk of hip fractures by 30 percent. The other two show *no effect* on preventing hip fractures.

- **Zometa or Reclast (zoledronic acid).** No meta-analyses have been done. Just three prospective trials involving up to 3,889 people and lasting up to three years. Zometa/Reclast cut the risk of vertebral fractures 67 percent and hip fractures 41 percent.

- **Aredia (pamidronate).** No meta-analyses have been conducted. Very few studies. Aredia appears to reduce vertebral fracture risk about 33 percent. Its effect against hip fractures, if any, is not known.

Most of the bisphosphonates come in tablets taken by mouth: Fosamax (alendronate), Actonel (risedronate), and Didronel (etidronate). Two must be injected: Aredia (pamidronate) daily and Zometa or Reclast (zoledronic acid) annually. One, Boniva (ibandronate), may be taken orally or by injection.

The oral bisphosphonates are absorbed poorly in the digestive tract. To maximize absorption, they must be taken on an empty stomach. Users are advised to take these drugs first thing in the morning with eight ounces of water and then not lie down or eat anything for at least thirty minutes.

The oral bisphosphonates may irritate the stomach and the esophagus, the tube from the throat into the stomach. Irritation may be minor, but in some cases painful esophageal ulcers develop.

The bisphosphonates work best when combined with supplemental calcium and vitamin D. In other words, for maximum benefit, users must take several pills daily, even if the drug is injected.

The bisphosphonates may also cause abdominal pain, muscle and joint pains, and, rarely, deterioration of the jawbone.

Forteo (Teriparatide)

Forteo is a genetically engineered version of parathyroid hormone, which promotes bone building. Forteo stimulates the osteoblasts to create bone.

Two meta-analyses and a few other studies show that Forteo reduces the risk of vertebral fractures by about 70 percent and the risk of hip, arm, and wrist fractures by about 50 percent.

The longest studies to date have tracked Forteo's effects for only two years. Until longer trial results are published, doctors are advised not to continue treatment past twenty-four months.

Forteo's side effects include muscle cramps, headache, nausea, dizziness, and abnormally high blood levels of calcium (hypercalcemia), which, in rare cases, is potentially fatal.

Forteo must be injected daily. Users do this themselves, like people with diabetes who inject insulin. Some people can't manage this and prefer oral medication.

Evista (Raloxifene)

Evista is similar to estrogen. It's not the hormone. It's a selective estrogen receptor modulator. It has some estrogenic effects and some antiestrogen action. Like the hormone, it suppresses osteoclast activity.

Five meta-analyses show that Evista reduces the risk of vertebral fractures approximately 40 percent. But it has little or no effect on hip fracture risk, at most a 10 percent decrease.

Unlike HRT, Evista does not increase the risk of heart disease, stroke, or breast cancer. However, it increases the risk of hot flashes and pulmonary embolism and triples the risk of other potentially serious internal blood clots (thromboembolism).

Miacalcin or Fortical (Calcitonin)

Miacalcin suppresses bone clearing by osteoclasts.

Three meta-analyses of up to 30 studies show widely varying results. For vertebral fractures, Miacalcin reduces risk 21 to 54 percent. But most of the studies are small. The largest one shows a risk reduction of only 21 percent. Nonvertebral fractures show the same disparate results. Miacalcin reduces the risk of hip, arm, and wrist fractures an average of 48 percent. But the one large study shows risk reduced by only 20 percent.

Miacalcin may be administered by injection or nasal spray. Fortical is a nasal spray.

The main side effect of the nasal spray is nasal irritation and congestion. Other side effects include stomach upset.

Americans Love Pills—or Do They?

When presented with a choice between taking pills and making diet and lifestyle changes, some people happily change their lives. But many others, perhaps most, would rather not make changes. They prefer drugs.

This makes sense. It's easier to pop a pill than change one's diet or begin an exercise program, even one as modest as walking thirty minutes a day. Hence the popular perception that "Americans love pills." But this adage obscures a greater truth: *many Americans do not take their medicine.*

Doctors wring their hands about medication "noncompliance." People get prescriptions but don't fill them. When they do, they don't take the drug as prescribed. Or they stop taking the medication before they should. Or they don't refill their prescriptions.

We found eight studies that track compliance with osteoporosis medications. Highlights:

- Researchers with Aetna, the health insurer, followed 10,566 people taking bisphosphonates for one year. Only 20 percent took the medication properly.
- For one year, Dutch researchers followed 2,124 women prescribed bisphosphonates. Among those taking one pill a week, only half (52 percent) kept it up for the full year. Among those taking a pill a day, only one-third (36 percent) continued all year.
- Columbia University researchers used health insurer databases to see how many of 35,537 women prescribed bisphosphonates refilled their prescriptions as one would expect if they took the medication as directed. Over a two-year period, only 20 percent had a refill pattern that suggested full compliance.
- A Yale meta-analysis of fourteen studies showed one-year bisphosphonate compliance varying from a low of 14 percent—

> just one person in seven—to a high of 78 percent. On average, about half the people took the drugs as prescribed.

No wonder the Aetna researchers called osteoporosis medication compliance "poor."

Actually, compliance is even worse. For maximum effectiveness, anyone taking an osteoporosis drug should also take calcium and vitamin D daily—meaning more pills and more lapses in taking them. University of North Carolina researchers surveyed people taking bisphosphonates. Only 59 percent took calcium, and just 45 percent took vitamin D.

Only about half of people take osteoporosis drugs as directed. And only around half chase them with the recommended calcium and vitamin D. So how effective are the osteoporosis drugs really? Less effective than the clinical trials and meta-analyses suggest.

The Most Cost-Effective Osteoporosis Drug

The three most effective osteoporosis drugs are Fosamax (alendronate), Forteo (teriparatide), and Zometa or Reclast (zoledronic acid).

All three drugs appear to be in the same ballpark in terms of effectiveness. They reduce hip fractures 40 to 50 percent.

Both Fosamax and Zometa/Reclast cost around $1,000 a year wholesale. Forteo costs *seven to ten times as much*, so it's nowhere near as cost-effective. Scratch Forteo.

Fosamax is a pill. Only about half of the people who receive prescriptions take it consistently as directed or take calcium and vitamin D along with it. Compliance problems sink it.

That leaves Zometa/Reclast. It's injected once a year at a doctor's office, so compliance is much less of an issue (though users may or may not take calcium and vitamin D as they should).

Assuming that future research corroborates the few studies we have, in our view, Zometa/Reclast (zoledronic acid) is the most cost-effective drug. It costs the same as Fosamax but works better because compliance is less of an issue.

For Many, Thiazide Diuretics May Be Preferable to Osteoporosis Drugs

Beyond the drugs developed to combat osteoporosis, one class of blood pressure medication prevents fractures almost as well: thiazide diuretics, aka water pills (Diuril, chlorothiazide, hydrochlorothiazide, chlorthalidone, etc.). In addition, thiazides also reduce risk of heart disease and stroke, conditions that are highly prevalent in those at high risk for fracture.

The thiazides increase urination. They also decrease excretion of calcium in urine.

In people who are not diabetic, thiazides are the only first-line class of medication for high blood pressure. Millions of people take them—and might be able to save the expense and side effects of the osteoporosis drugs.

We found fourteen studies of fracture risk in people taking thiazides. Twelve (86 percent) show that these drugs reduce fractures 10 to 60 percent. In the largest prospective trials, thiazides cut fractures 30 percent:

- Dutch scientists tracked thiazide use and fractures in 7,891 older people for one year. Those who took a thiazide daily for the year suffered 54 percent fewer hip fractures.
- Researchers with the National Institute on Aging followed 9,518 elderly men for four years. Compared with those who did not take thiazides, users suffered 32 percent fewer hip fractures.
- Harvard researchers analyzed Nurses' Health Study data (83,728 women) during the ten years from 1982 to 1992. Compared with those who did not use thiazides, those who did suffered 22 percent fewer forearm fractures. Thiazide use for eight years or more reduced forearm fracture risk 37 percent and hip fracture risk 31 percent.
- In a meta-analysis, Australian researchers pooled the results of thirteen studies involving 29,600 people: "Thiazide users have a 20 percent reduction in fracture risk."

Thiazides increase urination considerably in those who eat a standard American high-salt diet. With lower salt/sodium intake, thiazides still increase urination, but less.

After taking thiazides, users must have easy access to a bathroom for several hours. Many other side effects are also possible, most of them mild, but some potentially serious. Reducing the dose usually eliminates them.

Thiazides have been around for a long time. Osteoporosis drugs have not been with us anywhere near as long. It's possible that over time new side effects will turn up for Fosamax et al. That's much less likely with thiazides.

For reasons that remain unclear, compliance is less of an issue with thiazides than osteoporosis drugs. We found five compliance studies. Results varied, but overall around 75 percent of people prescribed thiazides take them as directed—compared with just 50 percent for the osteoporosis drugs.

Best of all, thiazides are cheap. Really cheap. They cost only a small fraction of what the osteoporosis drugs cost. Doctors often prescribe them to the very people at greatest risk for fractures. Thiazides safely provide two important benefits with just one pill—for next to nothing.

However, to our knowledge, few doctors prescribe thiazides to simultaneously treat high blood pressure and fracture risk. We're not surprised. Thiazides are cheap and generic. No one makes big money from them. Therefore, drug companies have no incentive to tout their effectiveness in splashy advertising. As a result, most doctors remain in the dark about thiazides' dual utility. And so does the public.

The Bottom Line on Osteoporosis Drugs

Osteoporosis drugs (or thiazides) are likely to help those who truly need them, particularly people who have suffered osteoporotic fractures, frail nursing homes residents, and people with substantial bone loss for any reason. However, they are no cure for osteoporosis. If you already have substantial bone loss—very low BMD—you should work with your doctor to find the right medicine for you and take it as prescribed along with daily calcium and vitamin D supplements. In addition, you can still benefit from low-acid eating and daily walking.

But what about everyone else? Is it medically and fiscally wise to prescribe osteoporosis drugs to the millions of Americans with low bone mineral density? We think not.

The most cost-effective medications reduce fracture risk by about half (assuming good compliance plus daily calcium pills and vitamin D). But based on the research discussed in Chapters 7 and 13, low-acid eating and daily walking produce the same benefits—or greater benefits—more safely, for less money, and all the side effects are beneficial.

Recall the studies of hip fracture rates around the world. Quite a few countries have 60, 70, even 80 percent fewer hip fractures than the United States, the United Kingdom, and Scandinavia—considerably fewer fractures than even an optimistic assessment of what the drugs produce. Yet osteoporosis drugs have played virtually no role in the low fracture rates in Asia and Africa. The lowest-fracture countries have relied entirely on low-acid eating and daily exercise.

Of course, change is difficult. Even with their health at stake, many people refuse to change their lives. They don't quit smoking. They struggle to change how they eat. They remain glued to the sofa. And they may not take their medicine.

If people resist diet and lifestyle changes, and they also resist taking drugs, what can we do to reduce the staggering toll of osteoporosis? Consider the smoking story.

Quitting smoking is very hard. Tobacco is strongly addictive. Many people try to quit but can't. Most try to quit several times before they succeed. Yet, thanks to coordinated efforts by physicians, legislatures, health agencies, private nonprofits, and the media, millions of people have quit successfully. Over the past forty years the proportion of Americans who smoke has been cut by more than half. We believe that a similar mobilization could persuade Americans to cut out or cut down substantially on animal foods, eat grains moderately, and eat at least five daily servings of fruits and vegetables, preferably more.

While a small proportion of Americans are good candidates for osteoporosis medication, the best, safest, most cost-effective approach to fracture prevention is low-acid eating and daily walking.

A Study We'd Like to See: Fosamax vs. Nature's Osteoporosis "Pills"

Raisins look sort of like pills. Raisins are also one of the most alkaline foods. (See Table 7.1.) A couple handfuls of raisins neutralize the acid produced by most animal foods. We would like to see a study comparing bone mineral density and fractures in people taking Fosamax for a year or two with people munching a few handfuls of raisins or other dried fruits every day. Would nature's pills beat drug pills? We don't know. But we think it's quite possible. If so, then dried fruit might replace many osteoporosis medication prescriptions and save the U.S. health care system billions of dollars a year. We'd like to see the National Institutes of Health fund a study to find out.

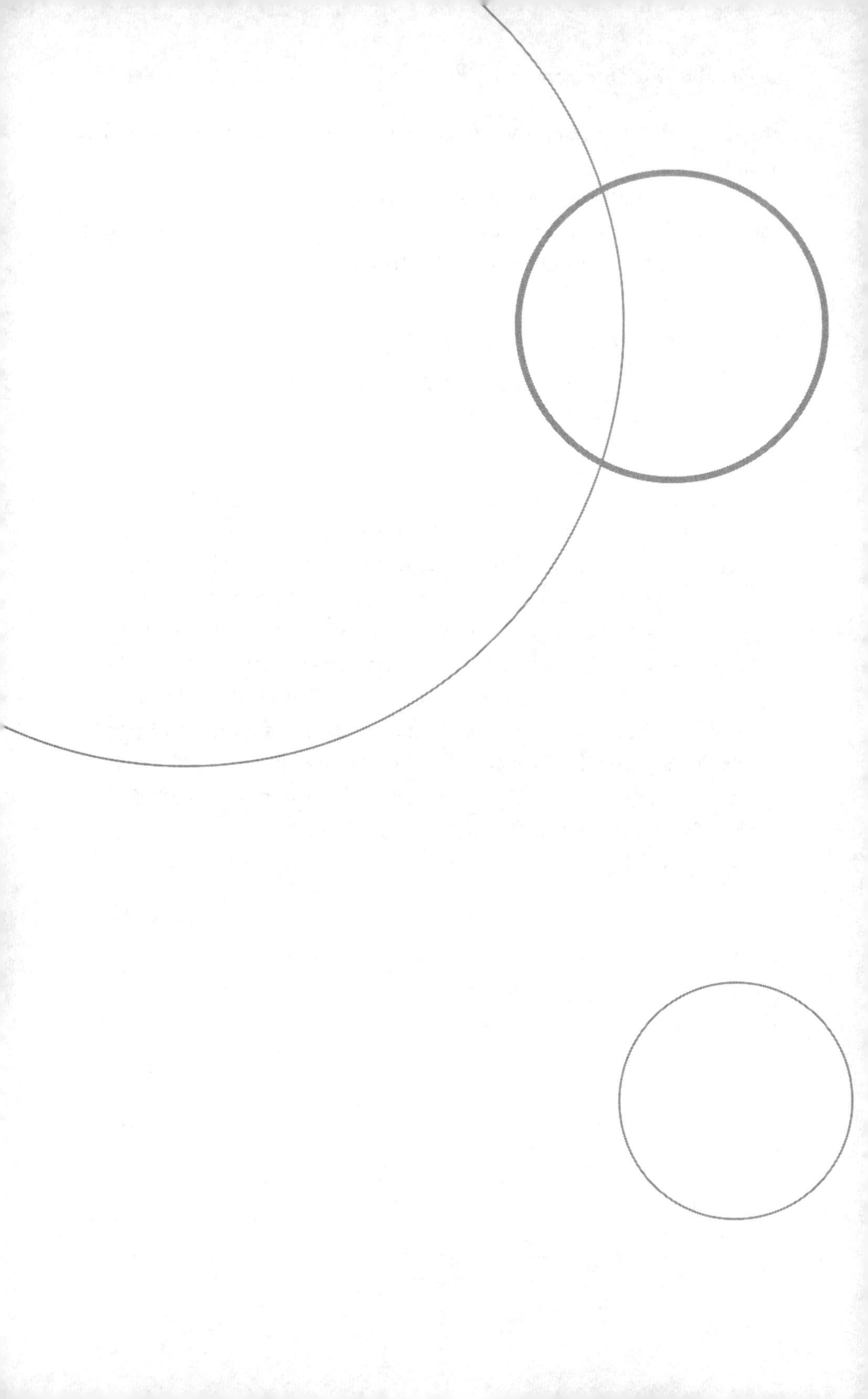

Save Your Bones and Save the Planet

In addition to substantially reducing the risk of fractures, heart disease, cancer, and other conditions, low-acid eating helps Mother Earth. Eating at least five servings of fruits and vegetables a day and consuming at most a few servings of animal foods a week substantially reduces petroleum use and the release of the greenhouse gases that cause global warming. It also prevents a great deal of soil erosion, air and water pollution, and loss of the tropical rain forests that create much of the planet's oxygen.

Recently the Food and Agriculture Organization of the United Nations (FAO) published a report, "Livestock's Long Shadow," that analyzes the worldwide environmental impact of the meat and dairy industries. The report concludes that cattle ranching and dairy farming make a "very substantial contribution to climate change, air pollution, and degradation of soil and water. The livestock sector is one of the top two or three most significant contributors to the most serious environmental problems at every level from local to global."

Highlights of the report:

- Cattle grazing occupies 26 percent of the planet's ice-free land, 33 percent of arable land worldwide, and 70 percent of all land devoted to agriculture. In other words, raising food animals uses more land than any other human activity.

- Expansion of livestock production causes deforestation, especially in Latin America, where the impact of deforestation is most severe. Compared with four hundred years ago, 70 percent of tropical rain forests in the Amazon have been deforested. Most of that land has been transformed into pastures for cattle grazing or fields for raising feed crops for livestock.

- An estimated 20 percent of the Earth's pastures and rangelands—and 73 percent of rangelands in dry areas—have been seriously degraded by soil erosion.

- Livestock production accounts for 18 percent of Earth-warming greenhouse gas production, a greater share than all motor vehicles—cars, trucks, buses, trains, ships, and planes—*combined*.

- When we burn petroleum fuels—gasoline, fuel oil, etc.—we add heat-trapping carbon dioxide to the atmosphere and the Earth gets warmer. As a result, the carbon footprint has become the focus of a great deal of media attention. But other gases play an even greater role in global warming. Compared with carbon dioxide, methane and nitrous oxide have respectively 23 times and 296 times more heat-trapping, global warming potential. The digestive processes of livestock release 37 percent of the methane and 65 percent of the nitrous oxide produced by human activity around the world.

- Cattle ranching and dairy farming also release almost two-thirds (64 percent) of human-produced ammonia, a gas that contributes significantly to acid rain and acidification of water supplies that kill fish and aquatic plants.

- Livestock (including poultry) produce more than a hundred times as much excrement as the entire U.S. human population, about forty-five tons (eighty-nine thousand pounds) per second.

- According to the Environmental Protection Agency, U.S. agriculture—much of it devoted to cattle ranching, dairy farming, and the production of feed crops—now accounts for nearly three-quarters of the water-quality problems in the nation's rivers and streams.

- Use of chemical fertilizers on feed crops is the world's largest contributor to water pollution. Fertilizers in agricultural water runoff—particularly compounds containing nitrogen or phosphorus—account for one-third of eutrophication, a process that causes explosive overgrowth of aquatic plants and deterioration of water quality. Fish and coral suffocate. You may have heard of the growing "dead zones" in the Gulf of Mexico and other areas near river mouths where fish can no longer be found. Blame eutrophication and the feed crop fertilizers that cause it.

- Erosion of pastureland and rangeland is responsible for more than half (55 percent) of sediments found in waterways and coastal areas.

- Cattle ranching and dairy farming account for 37 percent of pesticide use worldwide and 50 percent of antibiotic use. Pesticides in water runoff contribute to the decline of fish, seafood, and amphibian populations and to reproductive problems in the birds and other animals that eat them. Antibiotics used in livestock production contribute to the evolution of antibiotic-resistant bacteria.

- Meat and dairy cattle currently inhabit approximately 30 percent of the planet's ice-free land area. That figure is increasing. As more land is devoted to livestock, the species that once lived in those areas get pushed toward extinction. UN analysts estimate that the rate of extinctions is currently more than fifty times greater than the rate found in most of the fossil record. Livestock may well be the number-one cause of reduced biodiversity. The Worldwide Fund for Nature has identified 825 ecoregions around the world and reports that 306 of them (37 percent) face significant degradation from livestock production. Conservation International focuses on thirty-five global hot spots where biodiversity is significantly threatened. In twenty-three of them (66 percent), livestock production plays a major role in habitat loss.

- To produce one serving of beef, cattle ranchers use sixteen times as much gasoline as it takes to grow one serving of most vegetables.

- The land required to produce one serving of meat can produce approximately three servings of fruits and vegetables.

You can take a major step toward reducing your carbon footprint, minimizing greenhouse gases, and reversing erosion, eutrophication, and air and water pollution by embracing low-acid eating. Go vegetarian or at least eat fewer animal foods and more fruits and vegetables. Currently, Americans consume more than 220 pounds of meat per year. That's about ten ounces a day, 2.5 servings. If we reduced our meat consumption by just 20 percent—three fewer meat meals a week—this change would reduce the U.S. carbon footprint by as much as replacing all motor vehicles with ultraefficient hybrids.

By substantially reducing consumption of animal foods or eliminating them, low-acid eating reduces petroleum use, minimizes carbon footprint, and eliminates a great deal of greenhouse gases, soil erosion, air and water pollution, and habitat destruction. Low-acid eating allows us to reforest the Earth and still have plenty of land available to grow plant foods for a growing population and for production of plant-based fuels (ethanol, biodiesel, etc.). Low-acid eating not only saves bones. It saves the planet.

18

Conclusion: We Need an Evidence-Based Approach to Bone Vitality

Twenty-first century medicine strives to be evidence-based. No more treating conditions the way past generations of physicians have treated them simply because of tradition. Twenty-first century medicine demands compelling evidence that recommended treatments actually work.

We applaud this commitment to scientific rigor. We just wish our health authorities would apply it to osteoporosis.

The evidence is clear. Milk, dairy foods, and calcium pills don't strengthen bone or prevent fractures. What works is low-acid eating and walking or equivalent exercise for at least thirty minutes a day.

To be compelling, a scientific theory must work on many levels. Low-acid eating and daily walking work on six levels:

Epidemiology

The countries that consume the most calcium suffer the most fractures. Countries that consume little or no milk, dairy, and calcium pills suffer the fewest fractures—rates often 70 percent below those in the United

States, Western Europe, Scandinavia, Australia, and New Zealand. The conventional wisdom cannot explain this. The low-acid theory can.

Four large epidemiological surveys all show that as the amount of animal protein in the diet increases, so does the rate of hip fractures. And as the amount of vegetable protein rises, hip fractures fall. Using standard statistical techniques, these studies produce clear dose-response relationships, a hallmark of cause and effect.

The Mechanism of Action

Defenders of the conventional wisdom can't explain the epidemiology. They scratch their heads and mumble about the "calcium paradox." Only there is no paradox. The low-acid theory offers an elegant explanation for what we see around the world.

Like all animal foods, milk and dairy foods contain a great deal of protein. Digestion breaks it into amino acids. These acids enter the bloodstream and acidify the blood. Milk, dairy foods, and other animal foods do not contain enough alkaline material to buffer all this acid. To maintain the blood's pH in the narrow normal range, the body reaches into its alkaline reservoir, the calcium compounds in bone.

In addition, it takes more than calcium to build strong bones. It takes seventeen other nutrients. Milk, dairy, other animal foods, and calcium pills, even with added vitamin D, do not contain enough of these other nutrients to strengthen bones and keep them from fracturing. Fruits and vegetables do.

Fruits and vegetables contain small amounts of protein (but enough to meet the body's needs) buffered by large amounts of alkaline material. The amino acids in fruits and vegetables do not acidify the blood because, overall, fruits and vegetables are alkaline. Eat a plant-based diet, with a minimum of animal foods, if any, and the body has no need to suck calcium from bone.

Clinical Trials

How do diets high in animal foods or high in plant foods affect fracture rates? Eighteen studies published since 1975 have investigated this. Four (22 percent) show that a diet high in animal foods reduces fractures. Fourteen trials (78 percent) show that low-acid eating reduces fracture risk. The evidence supports the low-acid theory by almost four to one.

Cellular Level

When the blood's pH falls, as it becomes more acidic, bone-building osteoblasts are suppressed and bone-clearing osteoclasts go into overdrive. Meanwhile, optimally alkaline blood stimulates osteoblasts and suppresses osteoclasts. The conventional wisdom offers no insights into why this happens. The low-acid theory offers an elegant explanation.

When a diet high in animal foods makes the blood more acidic, the body directs the osteoclasts to chip away at bone and release calcium to neutralize the acid and return the blood to optimal pH. The body also quiets the osteoblasts because maintaining normal blood pH is more important to immediate survival than building new bone.

At the cellular level, a diet high in animal foods stimulates bone loss. A diet based on fruits and vegetables with a minimum of animal foods stimulates bone building.

Evolution

To believe the calcium theory, you have to believe that people have been drinking milk and eating cheese and yogurt forever. Otherwise, how could they grow strong bones? But like other mammals, for the vast majority of human evolution, our ancestors consumed little or no milk after weaning and no dairy foods. They couldn't digest milk sugar, lactose. The mutation that allows some of us to digest lactose occurred only about ten thousand years ago. Defenders of the calcium theory cannot explain how our preagricultural ancestors developed strong bones without milk and dairy foods. They generally say: Well, back then people didn't live long enough to develop osteoporosis. But some people did. Anthropological studies of the last remaining hunter-gatherer groups show that elders in those societies did not develop chronic disease, including osteoporosis, at anywhere near the rate of today's Americans.

The low-acid theory dovetails neatly with our understanding of human evolution. We humans evolved over some thirty million years from apelike creatures that subsisted largely on fruits, vegetables, nuts, and seeds. They ate meat only occasionally and no milk after weaning. Their bones grew strong and stayed strong because they ate a low-acid diet and walked a great deal to find the plant foods they ate. Meats, fish, milk, and grains became staples only ten thousand years ago. They supplied concentrated calories that reduced starvation and allowed humans to populate the Earth. But they led to chronically low-pH blood and osteoporosis (not to mention heart disease and many cancers). Our Stone Age bodies can't cope with our Space Age diet.

Biological Elegance

Anything that's beneficial to one system of an organism is almost always beneficial to everything else. Consider exercise. It reduces risk of obesity, anxiety, insomnia, diabetes, constipation, arthritis, stroke, sex problems, high cholesterol, high blood pressure, heart disease, many cancers, Alzheimer's disease—and osteoporosis. If milk and dairy build bone, they violate the principle of biological elegance. A diet high in whole milk and whole-milk dairy foods contains a great deal of saturated fat, and a mountain of research links saturated fat to increased risk of many of the conditions just mentioned.

In contrast, the low-acid theory is biologically elegant. The program we recommend for bone vitality—low-acid eating and daily walking—is the exact same program that health authorities recommend to reduce risk of obesity, diabetes, high cholesterol, high blood pressure, heart disease, stroke, cancer, Alzheimer's disease, and many other conditions.

How you live your life is up to you. If you want to eat 220 pounds of meat a year and only two to three servings of fruits and vegetables a day, you're free to do so. If you'd rather not be physically active, that's also your decision. But those decisions carry a high price—substantial risk of osteoporosis and our top causes of death: heart disease, cancer, and stroke.

If you want to cut your risk of osteoporosis by more than half and at the same time substantially reduce your risk of what kills twenty-first century Americans:

- Have two servings of fruit and/or vegetables at every meal and snack on fruit and vegetables.
- Cut down on—or eliminate—animal foods and go easy on cereals, breads, and pastas.
- Walk for at least a half hour a day from childhood to old age.

Low-acid eating and daily walking. They are the osteoporosis cure—and a safe, effective, low-cost prescription for health, vitality, and longevity.

Appendix A

Scorecard: Do Milk, Dairy Foods, and Calcium Supplements, by Themselves or Combined, Reduce the Risk of Fractures?

The twenty-four studies showing that they do:

1. Bischoff-Ferrari, H. A., et al. "Effect of Calcium Supplementation on Fracture Risk: A Double-Blind Randomized Trial." *American Journal of Clinical Nutrition* 87 (2008): 1945. Swiss researchers, University Hospital, Zurich. Calcium supplements. Prospective, 930 men and women over age 60 followed for 11 years. "Calcium supplementation reduced the risk of fractures."

2. Chan, H. H., et al. "Dietary Calcium Intake, Physical Activity, and the Risk of Vertebral Fracture in Chinese." *Osteoporosis International* 6 (1996): 228. University of Hong Kong researchers. Milk and dairy. Retrospective, 481 elderly women.

3. Chevalley, T., et al. "Effects of Calcium Supplements on Femoral Bone Mineral Density and Vertebral Fracture Rate in Vitamin-D-Replete Elderly

Patients." *Osteoporosis International* 4 (1994): 245. Researchers at the University Hospital of Geneva, Switzerland. Calcium supplements. Prospective, 93 elderly participants, average age 72, followed for 18 months.

4. Chu, S. P., et al. "Risk Factors for Proximal Humerus Fracture." *American Journal of Epidemiology* 160 (2004): 360. Stanford University researchers. Milk and dairy. Retrospective, 448 fracture cases, men and women aged 45 or older, 2,023 controls. "Low dietary calcium intake was associated with increased risk of fractures."

5. Clark, P., et al. "Risk Factors for Osteoporotic Hip Fractures in Mexicans." *Archives of Medical Research* 29 (1998): 253. Mexican researchers. Milk and dairy. Retrospective, 152 fracture cases, both sexes, age 45 or older, 143 controls.

6. Diez-Perez, A., et al. "Prediction of Absolute Risk of Non-Spinal Fractures Using Clinical Risk Factors and Heel Quantitative Ultrasound." *Osteoporosis International* 18 (2007): 629. Milk and dairy. Prospective, 5,201 participants followed for 3 years.

7. Fujiwara, S., et al. "Risk Factors for Hip Fracture in a Japanese Cohort." *Journal of Bone and Mineral Research* 12 (1997): 998. Researchers at the Radiation Effects Research Foundation, Hiroshima. Milk and dairy. Prospective, 4,573 adults followed for 13 years. Milk and dairy reduced fracture risk significantly—but "marginally."

8. Holbrook, T. L., et al. "Dietary Calcium and Risk of Hip Fracture: 14-Year Prospective Population Study." *Lancet* 2 (1988): 1046. UC San Diego researchers. Milk and dairy. Prospective, 957 men and women over age 50 followed for 14 years. Results "strongly support the hypothesis that increased dietary calcium intake protects against hip fracture."

9. Honkanen, R. J., et al. "Risk Factors for Perimenopausal Distal Forearm Fracture." *Osteoporosis International* 11 (2000): 265. Researchers at the University of Kuopio, Finland. Milk and dairy. Prospective, 11,798 participants followed for 5 years.

10. Kalkwarf, H. J., et al. "Milk Intake During Childhood and Adolescence, Adult Bone Density, and Osteoporotic Fractures in U.S. Women." *American Journal of Clinical Nutrition* 77 (2003): 257. Children's Hospital Medical Center, Cincinnati. Milk and dairy. Retrospective, 3,251 white women who, in many cases, recalled their milk consumptions over more than 50 years.

"Low milk intake during childhood was associated with a two-fold greater risk of hip fracture" later in life.

11. Kanis, J., et al. "Risk Factors for Hip Fracture in Men from Southern Europe: The MEDOS Study: Mediterranean Osteoporosis Study." *Osteoporosis International* 9 (1999): 45. Researchers at the University of Sheffield, England. Milk and dairy. Retrospective, 730 elderly men, 1,132 controls. While low intake of milk and cheese increased fracture risk significantly, fewer than 9 percent of fractures could be attributed to low milk and dairy consumption.

12. Kelsey, J. L., et al. "Risk Factors for Stress Fracture Among Young Female Cross-Country Runners." *Medicine and Science in Sports and Exercise* 39 (2007): 1457. Stanford University researchers. Milk and dairy. Prospective, 127 female runners, ages 18 to 26, followed for almost 2 years.

13. Kelsey, J. L., et al. "Reducing the Risk for Distal Forearm Fracture: Preserve Bone Mass, Slow Down, and Don't Fall." *Osteoporosis International* 16 (2005): 681. Stanford University researchers. Milk and dairy. Retrospective, 1,150 cases, 2,331 controls, all aged 45 or older.

14. Kung, A. W., et al. "Ten-Year Risk of Osteoporotic Fractures in Post-Menopausal Chinese Women According to Clinical Risk Factors and BMD T-Scores: A Prospective Study." *Journal of Bone and Mineral Research* 22 (2007): 1080. University of Hong Kong researchers. Milk and dairy. Prospective, 1,435 elderly women followed for 10 years.

15. Lau, E., et al. "Physical Activity and Calcium Intake in Fracture of the Proximal Femur in Hong Kong." *BMJ* [formerly *British Medical Journal*] 297 (6661) (1988): 1441. University of Hong Kong researchers. Milk and dairy. Retrospective, 400 cases, 800 controls. "High [calcium] intake protected against fractures."

16. Lumbers, M., et al. "Nutritional Status in Elderly Female Hip Fracture Patients: Comparison with and Age-Matched Home Living Group Attending Day Centers." *British Journal of Nutrition* 85 (2001): 733. British researchers at the University of Surrey. Milk and dairy. Retrospective, 75 cases, 50 controls, all elderly women.

17. Michael, B. A., et al. "Physical Activity and Fractures Over the Age of Fifty Years." *International Orthopedics* (1992) 16:87. Swiss researchers. Milk and dairy. Retrospective, 456 cases, 266 controls. "Men and women with a high calcium intake had fewer fractures."

18. Myburgh, K. H., et al. "Low Bone Density is an Etiological Factor for Stress Fractures in Athletes." *Annals of Internal Medicine* 113 (1990): 754. Researchers at the University of Cape Town Medical School, South Africa. Milk and dairy. Retrospective, 25 cases, 25 controls.

19. Nevitt, M. C., et al. "Risk Factors for a First-Incident Radiographic Vertebral Fracture in Women > or = 65 Years of Age: The Study of Osteoporotic Fractures." *Journal of Bone and Mineral Research* 20 (2005): 131. University of California, San Francisco, researchers. Milk and dairy. Prospective, 5,822 women aged 65 or older followed for 3.7 years.

20. Perez-Cano, R., et al. "Risk Factors for Hip Fracture in Spanish and Turkish Women." *Bone* 14 (Suppl 1) (1993): S69. Spanish researchers. Milk and dairy. Retrospective, 519 cases, women aged 50 or older, 808 controls.

21. Pires, L. A., et al. "Bone Mineral Density, Milk Intake, and Physical Activity in Boys Who Suffer Forearm Fractures." *Journal of Pediatrics (Rio de Janeiro)* 81 (2005): 332. Researchers from Universidade Federal do Rio Grande do Sul, Porto Allegre, Brazil. Milk and dairy. Retrospective, 23 cases, 23 controls.

22. Reid, I. R., et al. "Long-Term Effects of Calcium Supplementation on Bone Loss and Fractures in Postmenopausal Women: A Randomized Controlled Trial." *American Journal of Medicine* 98 (1995): 331. Researchers at the University of Auckland, New Zealand. Calcium supplements. Prospective, 78 elderly women followed for 4 years.

23. Tuppurainen, M., et al. "Osteoporosis Risk Factors, Gynecological History, and Fractures in Perimenopausal Women: Results of the Baseline Postal Enquiry of the Kuopio Osteoporosis Risk Factor and Prevention Study." *Maturitas* 17 (1993): 89. Finnish researchers. Milk and dairy. Retrospective, 13,196 women ages 47 to 56 surveyed.

24. Wyshak, G., and R. E. Frisch. "Carbonated Beverages, Dietary Calcium, the Dietary Calcium/Phosphorus Ratio, and Bone Fractures in Girls and Boys." *Journal of Adolescent Health* 15 (1994): 210. Harvard researchers. Milk and dairy. Retrospective, 76 girls, 51 boys, average age 14.

The fifteen inconclusive studies:

1. Center, J. R., et al. "Risk of Subsequent Fracture After Low-Trauma Fracture in Men and Women." *Journal of the American Medical Association* 297 (2007): 387. Australian researchers. Milk and dairy. Prospective, 4,005

elderly men and women followed for 16 years. High calcium intake reduced fractures in men but not women.

2. Cooper, C., et al. "Physical Activity, Muscle Strength, and Calcium Intake in Fracture of the Proximal Femur in Britain." *BMJ* [formerly *British Medical Journal*] 297 (6661) (1988): 1443. University of Southampton researchers. Milk and dairy. Retrospective, 300 cases, 600 controls. High calcium intake reduced fractures in men but not women.

3. Cumming, R. G., and M. C. Nevitt. "Calcium for Prevention of Osteoporotic Fractures in Postmenopausal Women." *Journal of Bone and Mineral Research* 12 (1997): 1321. Researchers at the University of Sydney, Australia. Meta-analysis of 37 milk and dairy studies. Findings "not consistent" and "not easily explained."

4. Honkanen, R., et al. "Lactose Intolerance Associated with Fracture of Weight-Bearing Bones in Finnish Women Aged 38–57 Years." *Bone* 21 (1997): 473. Researchers at the University of Tromso, Norway. Milk and dairy. Retrospective survey of 11,619 women. Lactose intolerance reduces milk and dairy intake and therefore calcium. Lactose-intolerant women had more fractures of the shinbone and bones in the foot. But lactose intolerance was not related to fractures of the wrist, ankle, or rib.

5. Huang, Z., et al. "Nutrition and Subsequent Hip Fracture Risk Among a National Cohort of White Women." *American Journal of Epidemiology* 144 (1996): 124. University of Minnesota researchers. Milk and dairy. Prospective, 2,513 women, aged 45 or older, followed for up to 5 years. "Although dietary calcium is assumed to be an important nutrient that influences bone mass and fracture risk, this study showed that dietary calcium was only marginally related to hip fracture risk."

6. Johnell, O., et al. "Risk Factors for Hip Fracture in European Women: The MEDOS Study, Mediterranean Osteoporosis Study." *Journal of Bone and Mineral Research* 10 (1995): 1802. Researchers at Malmo General Hospital, Sweden. Milk and dairy. Retrospective study of women over age 50 at 14 centers in Portugal, Spain, France, Italy, Greece, and Turkey. Fracture risk was elevated in only the 10 percent of women with the lowest milk intake and not in the other 90 percent of participants.

7. Kreiger, N., et al. "Dietary Factors and Fracture in Postmenopausal Women: A Case-Control Study." *International Journal of Epidemiology* 21 (1992): 953. Researchers from University of Toronto, Ontario, Canada.

Milk and dairy. Retrospective, 256 cases, 277 controls. High calcium intake reduced the risk of wrist fracture but *increased* the risk of hip fracture.

8. Kudlacek, S., et al. "Lactose Intolerance: A Risk Factor for Reduced Bone Mineral Density and Vertebral Fractures?" *Journal of Gastroenterology* 37 (2002): 1014. Austrian researchers in Vienna. Milk and dairy. Retrospective, 115 cases, 103 controls. Lactose-intolerant subjects had more vertebral fractures but no greater risk of other fractures (hip, wrist, ankle).

9. Looker, A. C., et al. "Dietary Calcium and Hip Fracture Risk: the NHANES I Epidemiologic Follow-Up Study." *Osteoporosis International* 3 (1993): 177. Milk and dairy. Prospective, 4,342 women, ages 50 to 74 at the start, followed for 16 years. Overall, dietary calcium made no difference to fracture risk. In the oldest women, calcium appeared protective, but the results were not statistically significant.

10. Matkovic, V., et al. "Bone Status and Fracture Rates in Two Regions of Yugoslavia." *American Journal of Clinical Nutrition* 52 (1979): 540. Milk and dairy. Retrospective. Fifty cases and controls from regions with high and low calcium intake. The low-calcium region had elevated risk of hip fracture but the same risk of forearm fracture.

11. Prince, R. L., et al. "Effects of Calcium Supplementation on Clinical Features and Bone Structure: Results of a Five-Year, Double-Blind, Placebo-Controlled Trial in Elderly Women." *Archives of Internal Medicine* 166 (2006): 869. University of Western Australia researchers. Calcium supplements. Prospective, 1,460 elderly women, average age 75, followed for 5 years. Overall, calcium supplements had no effect on fracture risk. But a subgroup experienced fewer fractures. The researchers concluded: "Supplementation with calcium is ineffective as a public health intervention for fracture prevention."

12. Recker, R. R., et al. "Correcting Calcium Nutritional Deficiency Prevents Spine Fractures in Elderly Women." *Journal of Bone and Mineral Research* 11 (1996): 1961. Creighton University researchers. Milk, dairy, and calcium supplements combined. Prospective, 197 women over age 60 at the start, followed for 4.3 years. Calcium did not reduce fracture risk in women with no previous fracture. It did reduce risk in those with a previous fracture.

13. Reid, I. R., et al. "Randomized Controlled Trial of Calcium in Healthy Older Women." *American Journal of Medicine* 119 (2006): 777. New Zea-

land researchers. Calcium supplements. Prospective, 1,471 women aged 70 or older followed for 5 years. "Calcium results in a sustained reduction in bone loss, but its effect on fracture remains uncertain."

14. Shea, B., et al. "Calcium Supplementation on Bone Loss in Postmenopausal Women." *Cochrane Database Systematic Review* CD004526 (2004). International group of researchers. This meta-analysis of calcium supplements shows a trend toward fracture reduction, but the results were not statistically significant. This same meta-analysis was published in *Endocrinology Reviews* 23 (2002): 552.

15. Yaegashi, Y., et al. "Association of Hip Fracture Incidence and Intake of Calcium, Magnesium, Vitamin D, and Vitamin K." *European Journal of Epidemiology* 23 (2008): 219. Japanese researchers. Milk and dairy. Retrospective, estimates of cases from 12 regional medical centers. Controls based on population surveys. Calcium intake reduced fractures in women but not men.

The forty-seven studies showing that milk and dairy foods do not reduce risk of fractures:

1. Albrand, G., et al. "Independent Predictors of All Osteoporosis-Related Fractures in Healthy Postmenopausal Women: the OFELY Study." *Bone* 32 (2003): 78. Researchers at the University of Lyon, France. Milk, dairy, and calcium supplements combined. Prospective, 672 postmenopausal women followed for 5.3 years. Calcium intake did not predict fracture risk.

2. Almustafa, M., et al. "Effects of Treatments by Calcium and Sex Hormones on Vertebral Fracturing in Osteoporosis." *QJM* [*Quarterly Journal of Medicine*] 83 (1992): 283. British researchers. Calcium supplements. Prospective, 49 women followed for 3 years. "Both postmenopausal and nonmenopausal women who did not receive sex hormones failed to show a reduction in fracture on high calcium alone."

3. Bischoff-Ferrari, H. A., et al. "Calcium Intake and Hip Fracture Risk in Men and Women: A Meta-Analysis of Prospective Cohort Studies and Randomized Controlled Trials." *American Journal of Clinical Nutrition* 86 (2007): 1780. Harvard researchers. Meta-analysis of 7 milk and dairy trials involving 170,991 women. "There was no association between total calcium intake and hip fracture risk."

4. Campbell, I. A., et al. "Five-Year Study of Etidronate and/or Calcium as Prevention and Treatment for Osteoporosis and Fractures in Patients with

Asthma Receiving Longterm Oral and/or Inhaled Glucocorticoids." *Thorax* 59 (2004): 761. British researchers. Calcium supplements. Prospective, 349 postmenopausal women followed for 5 years. "The effects of calcium were not significant."

5. Cumming, R. G., et al. "Case-Control Study of Risk Factors for Hip Fractures in the Elderly." *American Journal of Epidemiology* 139 (1994): 493. Researchers at the University of Sydney, Australia. Milk and dairy. Retrospective, 209 cases, 207 controls over age 65. Those who consumed the most milk and dairy at age 20 had *increased risk* of fracture after age 65—*almost triple the average risk.*

6. Cumming, R. G., et al. "Calcium Intake and Fracture Risk: Results from the Study of Osteoporotic Fractures." *American Journal of Epidemiology* 145 (1997): 926. Researchers at the University of Sydney, Australia. Milk, dairy, and calcium supplements combined. Prospective, 9,704 elderly women followed for an average of 6.6 years. As calcium intake from supplements rose, fracture risk *increased*. "This study did not find a substantial beneficial effect of calcium on fracture risk."

7. Cummings, S. R., et al. "Risk Factors for Hip Fracture in White Women. Study of Osteoporotic Fractures Research Group." *New England Journal of Medicine* 332 (1995): 767. Researchers at the University of California, San Francisco. Milk and dairy. Prospective, 9,516 elderly women followed for 4 years. Dietary calcium was unrelated to fracture risk.

8. Farmer, M. E., et al. "Anthropometric Indicators and Hip Fracture: The NHANES I Epidemiologic Follow-Up Study." *Journal of the American Geriatric Society* 37 (1989): 9. NHANES is the National Health and Nutrition Examination Survey, a project of the Centers for Disease Control and Prevention (CDC) that tracks American diet and health. Milk and dairy. Prospective, 3,595 women, ages 40 to 77 at the start, followed for 10 years. Calcium consumption made no difference to fracture risk.

9. Feskanich, D., et al. "Milk, Dietary Calcium, and Bone Fractures in Women: A 12-Year Prospective Study." *American Journal of Public Health* 87 (1997): 992. Harvard researchers. Milk and dairy. Prospective, 77,761 women, ages 34 to 59 at the start, followed for 12 years. Compared with women who drank one glass of milk or less per week, those who drank two or more glasses had *greater risk* of hip fracture.

10. Feskanich, D., et al. "Calcium, Vitamin D, Milk Consumption, and Hip Fractures: A Prospective Study Among Postmenopausal Women." *American Journal of Clinical Nutrition* 77 (2003): 504. Harvard researchers. Milk, dairy, and calcium supplements combined. Prospective, 72,337 older women followed for 18 years. "Neither milk nor a high-calcium diet appears to reduce [fracture] risk."

11. Grant, A. M., et al. "Oral Vitamin D3 and Calcium for Secondary Prevention of Low-Trauma Fractures in Elderly People (Randomized Evaluation of Calcium or Vitamin D, the RECORD study): A Randomized, Placebo-Controlled Trial." *Lancet* 365 (9471) (2005): 1621. Researchers at the University of Aberdeen, Scotland. Calcium supplements. Prospective, 5,292 participants, aged 70 or older, followed for up to 5 years. "The incidence of new fractures did not differ significantly between participants allocated calcium and those who were not."

12. Hagino, H., et al. "Case-Control Study of Risk Factors for Fractures of the Distal Radius and Proximal Humerus Among the Japanese Population." *Osteoporosis International* 15 (2004): 226. Japanese researchers. Milk and dairy. Retrospective, 140 cases, 242 controls, all women over 45. "There was no significant correlation with milk to the risk of either fracture."

13. Huopio, J., et al. "Risk Factors for Perimenopausal Fractures: A Prospective Study." *Osteoporosis International* 11 (2000): 219. Kuopio University researchers, Finland. Milk and dairy. Prospective, 3,068 women, ages 47 to 56 at the start, followed for 3.6 years. "Dietary calcium intake was not independently associated with any type of fracture."

14. Jonsson, B., et al. "Lifestyle and Different Fracture Prevalence: A Cross-Sectional Comparative Population-Based Study." *Calcified Tissue International* 52 (1993): 425. Swedish reseachers Milk and dairy. Retrospective, comparing 782 urban dwellers with 486 rural. Urban residents had higher fractures rates. Less weight-bearing exercise explained the difference. Calcium intake had no impact.

15. Kanis, J. A., et al. "A Meta-Analysis of Milk Intake and Fracture Risk: Low Utility for Case Finding." *Osteoporosis International* 16 (2005): 799. Meta-analysis of six milk and dairy prospective trials with a total of 39,563 participants followed for an average of 3.8 years. "No significant relationship was observed for low milk intake and hip fracture risk."

16. Kato, I., et al. "Diet, Smoking, and Anthropometric Indices and Postmenopausal Bone Fractures: A Prospective Study." *International Journal of Epidemiology* 29 (2000): 85. New York University researchers. Milk and dairy. Prospective, 6,250 postmenopausal women followed for 7.6 years. "The majority of epidemiological studies, including this one, have not shown that higher calcium intake within usual dietary levels is protective against osteoporotic fractures."

17. Kawada, T. "Factors Influencing Bone Fractures in Severely Disabled Persons." *American Journal of Physical Medicine and Rehabilitation* 81 (2002): 424. Japanese researcher. Milk and dairy. Retrospective, 73 cases, 73 controls. Calcium intake was not significantly related to fracture risk.

18. Kelsey, J. L., et al. "Risk Factors for Fracture of the Distal Forearm and Proximal Humerus. The Study of Osteoporotic Fractures Research Group." *American Journal of Epidemiology* 135 (1992): 477. Stanford University researchers. Milk and dairy. Prospective, 9,704 elderly women followed for 2.2 years. Dietary calcium was unrelated to fracture risk.

19. Kelsey, J. L., et al. "Risk Factors for Fracture of the Shafts of the Tibia and Fibula in Older Individuals." *Osteoporosis International* 17 (2006): 143. Stanford University researchers. Milk, dairy, and calcium supplements combined. Retrospective, 179 cases, 2,399 controls. "Higher dietary calcium intake and use of calcium supplements, which would be expected to be associated with higher bone mass, did not have much effect on [fracture] risk."

20. Kleerekoper, M., et al. "Identification of Women at Risk for Developing Postmenopausal Osteoporosis with Vertebral Fractures: Role of History and Single Photon Absorptiometry." *Bone Mineralization* 7 (1989): 171. Researchers at Henry Ford Hospital, Detroit, Michigan. Milk, dairy, and calcium supplements combined. Retrospective, 266 cases, 397 controls. Fracture cases and nonfractured controls "did not differ with respect to dietary intake of milk, cheese or calcium supplements."

21. Korpelainen, R., et al. "Lifelong Risk Factors for Osteoporosis and Fractures in Elderly Women with Low Body Mass Index: A Population-Based Study." *Bone* 39 (2006): 385. Finnish researchers. Milk and dairy. Retrospective, 1,222 elderly women surveyed. Calcium intake had no effect on fracture risk.

22. La Vecchia, C., et al. "Cigarette Smoking, Body Mass, and Other Risk Factors for Fractures of the Hip in Women." *International Journal of Epidemiology* 20 (1991): 671. Italian researchers. Milk and dairy. Retrospective, 209 cases, 1,449 controls. "Aspects of diet were investigated, including such important sources of calcium as milk, cheese, and butter. None of these was related to hip fracture."

23. Loud, K. J., et al. "Correlates of Stress Fractures Among Preadolescent and Adolescent Girls." *Pediatrics* 115 (2005): e399. Harvard researchers. Milk, dairy, and calcium supplements combined. Retrospective, 5,461 girls, average age 14. "Calcium intake and daily dairy intake were all unrelated to stress fractures."

24. Ma, D., and G. Jones. "Soft Drink and Milk Consumption, Physical Activity, Bone Mass, and Upper Limb Fractures in Children: A Population-Based, Case-Control Study." *Calcified Tissues International* 75 (2004): 286. Australian researchers. Milk and dairy. Retrospective, 206 cases, 206 controls. Average weekly milk consumption had no effect on fracture risk.

25. Meyer, H. E., et al. "Dietary Factors and Incidence of Hip Fracture in Middle-Aged Norwegians: A Prospective Study." *American Journal of Epidemiology* 145 (1997): 117. National Health Service researchers, Oslo, Norway. Milk and dairy. Prospective, 19,752 women, 20,035 men, ages 37 to 52 at the start, followed for 11.4 years. "There was no clear association between calcium intake and hip fracture."

26. Meyer, H. E., et al. "Risk Factors for Femoral Neck Fractures in Oslo." *Tidsskr. Nor. Laeeforen.* [Norwegian journal] 116 (1996): 2656. Norwegian researchers. Retrospective, 246 cases, 246 controls. "We found no relation between calcium intake and hip fracture."

27. Meyer, H. E., et al. "Risk Factors for Hip Fracture in a High-Incidence Area: A Case-Control Study from Oslo, Norway." *Osteoporosis International* 5 (1995): 239. University of Oslo researchers. Milk and dairy. Retrospective, 246 cases, 246 controls. With regard to hip fracture risk, "no association with dietary calcium intake was found."

28. Michaelsson, K., et al. "Dietary Calcium and Vitamin D in Relation to Osteoporotic Fracture Risk." *Bone* 32 (2003): 694. Researchers from the University of Uppsala, Sweden. Milk and dairy. Prospective, 60,689 women,

ages 40 to 74 at the start, followed for 11 years. "We found no dose-response association between dietary calcium intake and fracture risk."

29. Michaelsson, K., et al. "Diet and Hip Fracture Risk: A Case-Control Study. Study Group of the Multiple Risk Survey on Swedish Women for Eating Assessment." *International Journal of Epidemiology* 24 (1995): 771. Researchers at Central Hospital, Vasteras, Sweden. Milk and dairy. Retrospective, 247 cases, 893 controls. "High calcium intake did not protect against hip fracture."

30. Mussolino, M. E., et al. "Risk Factors for Hip Fracture in White Men: the NHANES I Epidemiologic Follow-Up Study." *Journal of Bone and Mineral Research* 13 (1998): 918. Researchers with the Centers for Disease Control and Prevention. Milk and dairy. Prospective, 2,879 adults, ages 45 to 74, followed for 22 years. Milk and dairy intake was not significantly related to fracture risk.

31. Nguyen, T. V., et al. "Risk Factors for Osteoporotic Fractures in Elderly Men." *American Journal of Epidemiology* 144 (1996): 255. Australian researchers. Milk and dairy. Prospective, 220 men over 60 followed for 5 years.

32. Nieves, J. W., et al. "A Case-Control Study of Hip Fracture: Evaluation of Selected Dietary Variables and Teenage Physical Activity." *Osteoporosis International* 2 (1992): 122. Columbia University researchers. Milk and dairy. Retrospective study, 161 elderly women cases, 168 age-matched controls. "No association was found between intake of calcium and hip fracture."

33. O'Neill, T. W., et al. "Risk Factors, Falls, and Fracture of the Distal Forearm in Manchester, UK." *Journal of Epidemiology and Community Health* 50 (1996): 288. British researchers. Milk and dairy. Retrospective, 62 cases, 166 controls. "Calcium intake was not associated with fracture."

34. Owusu, W., et al. "Calcium Intake and Incidence of Forearm and Hip Fractures Among Men." *Journal of Nutrition* 127 (1997): 1782. Harvard researchers. Milk, dairy, and calcium supplements combined. Prospective, 43,063 men over 40 followed for 8 years. "These results do not support a relation between calcium intake and incidence of fractures in men."

35. Paganini-Hill, A., et al. "Menopausal Estrogen Therapy and Hip Fractures." *Annals of Internal Medicine* 95 (1981): 28. University of Southern California researchers. Calcium supplements. Retrospective, 91 cases, 80 controls.

36. Paganini-Hill, A., et al. "Exercise and Other Factors in the Prevention of Hip Fracture: The Leisure World Study." *Epidemiology* 2 (1991): 16. University of Southern California researchers. Milk, dairy, and calcium supplements combined. Prospective, 13,649 elderly men and women followed for 7 years.

37. Petridou, E., et al. "The Role of Dairy Products and Non-Alcoholic Beverages in Bone Fractures Among Schoolage Children." *Scandinavian Journal of Social Medicine* 25 (1997): 119. Athens University researchers, Greece. Milk and dairy. Retrospective, 100 cases (boys and girls), 100 age- and gender-matched controls. "Intake of dairy products was not related to the occurrence of fractures."

38. Ramalho, A. C., et al. "Osteoporotic Fractures of the Proximal Femur: Clinical and Epidemiological Features in a Population of the City of Sao Paulo." *Sao Paulo Medical Journal* 119 (2001): 48. Milk and dairy. Retrospective, elderly men and women, 73 cases, 73 matched controls. Calcium intake was unrelated to fracture risk.

39. Ribot, C., and J. M. Pouilles. "Postmenopausal Osteoporosis: Clinical Characteristics in Patients' First Vertebral Crush Fracture. Results of the GRIO National Multicenter Survey. Groupe de Recherche et d'Information sure les Osteoporoses." *Review of Rheumatology Education, France* 60 (1993): 427. French researchers. Milk and dairy. Retrospective, 74 cases, 74 controls. Calcium intake "was similar in the two groups."

40. Robbins, J., et al. "Factors Associated with 5-Year Risk of Hip Fracture in Postmenopausal Women." *Journal of the American Medical Association* 298 (2007): 2389. Researchers at the University of California, at Davis. Milk, dairy, and calcium supplements combined. Prospective, 10,750 women followed for 7.6 years.

41. Roy, D. K., et al. "Determinants of Incident Vertebral Fracture in Men and Women: Results from the European Prospective Osteoporosis Study (EPOS)." *Osteoporosis International* 14 (2003): 19. British researchers. Milk and dairy. Prospective, 6,575 men and women, average age 62, followed for 3.8 years.

42. Tavani, A., et al. "Calcium, Dairy Products, and the Risk of Hip Fracture in Women in Northern Italy." *Epidemiology* 6 (1995): 554. Researchers at the University of Milan, Italy. Milk, dairy, and calcium supplements combined. Retrospective, 241 cases, 719 controls. "There was little asso-

ciation between hip fractures in women and intake of calcium, milk, and cheese."

43. Taylor, B. C., et al. "Long-Term Prediction of Incident Hip Fracture Risk in Elderly White Women: Study of Osteoporotic Fractures." *Journal of the American Geriatric Society* 52 (2004): 1479. University of Minnesota researchers. Calcium supplements. Prospective, 6,787 participants followed for 10 years.

44. Turner, L. W., et al. "Osteoporotic Fracture Among Older U.S. Women: Risk Factors Quantified." *Journal of Aging and Health* 10 (1998): 372. University of Arkansas researchers. Milk and dairy. Retrospective, 2,325 participants. As dairy intake increased, so did risk of hip fracture. Dietary calcium intake was not a risk factor for fractures.

45. Turner, L. W., et al. "Risk Factors for Hip Fracture Among Southern Older Women." *Southern Medical Journal* 91 (1998): 533. University of Arkansas researchers. Milk and dairy. Retrospective, 953 participants. Dairy product intake did not protect against fractures.

46. Valimaki, V. V., et al. "Risk Factors for Clinical Stress Fractures in Male Military Recruits: A Prospective Cohort Study." *Bone* 37 (2005): 267. Finnish researchers. Milk and dairy. Prospective, 179 men, ages 18 to 20, followed for 1 year. Calcium consumption was unrelated to fracture risk.

47. Wickham, C. A., et al. "Dietary Calcium, Physical Activity, and Risk of Hip Fracture: A Prospective Study." *BMJ* [formerly *British Medical Journal*] 299 (6704) (1989): 889. Milk and dairy. Prospective, 720 elderly men, 699 elderly women, followed for 15 years. "Reduced intake of dietary calcium did not seem to be a risk factor for hip fracture."

Appendix B
Scorecard: Do Milk, Dairy, and Calcium Intake During Childhood Prevent Fractures?

The two research reviews that say no:

1. Lanou, A. J., et al. "Calcium, Dairy Products, and Bone Health in Children and Young Adults: A Re-Evaluation of the Evidence." *Pediatrics* 115 (2005): 736. Conclusion: No benefit.

2. Winzenberg, T., et al. "Effects of Calcium Supplementation on Bone Density in Healthy Children: Meta-Analysis of Randomized Controlled Trials." *BMJ* [formerly *British Medical Journal*] 333 (7572) (2006): 775. Australian researchers. Conclusion: No benefit from calcium supplements.

The six studies showing that milk, dairy, and calcium intake during childhood reduce fracture risk during childhood and throughout life:

1. Kalkwarf, H. J., et al. "Milk Intake During Childhood and Adolescence, Adult Bone Density, and Osteoporotic Fractures in U.S. Women." *American Journal of Clinical Nutrition* 77 (2003): 257. Children's Hospital, Cincinnati, researchers. Retrospective, 3,251 white women. "Low milk intake during childhood was associated with a two-fold greater risk of fracture."

2. Manias, K., et al. "Fractures and Recurrent Fractures in Children: Varying Effects of Environmental Factors as Well as Bone Size and Mass." *Bone* 39 (2006): 652. British researchers. Retrospective, 150 children ages 4 to 16, 50 who had suffered 1 fracture, 50 who had suffered more than 1 fracture, and 50 fracture-free controls. "Children with recurrent fractures had a significantly lower milk intake."

3. Myburgh, K. H., et al. "Low Bone Density is an Etiologic Factor for Stress Fracture in Athletes." *Annals of Internal Medicine* 113 (1990): 754. South African researchers. Retrospective, 25 cases, 25 controls. "Athletes with fractures had lower calcium intakes."

4. Pires, L. A., et al. "Bone Mineral Density, Milk Intake and Physical Activity in Boys Who Suffer Forearm Fractures." *Journal of Pediatrics (Rio de Janeiro)* 81 (2005): 332. Brazilian researchers. Retrospective, 23 cases, 23 controls. "Milk intake was significantly lower in the case [fractured] group."

5. Wyshak, G., and R. E. Frisch. "Carbonated Beverages, Dietary Calcium, the Dietary Calcium/Phosphorus Ratio, and Bone Fracture in Girls and Boys." *Journal of Adolescent Health* 15 (1994): 210. Harvard researchers. Retrospective, 76 girls, 51 boys. "High intake of dairy calcium was protective [against fractures]."

6. Wyshak, G., et al. "Nonalcoholic Carbonated Beverage Consumption and Bone Fractures Among Women Former College Athletes." *Journal of Orthopedic Research* 7 (1989): 91. Harvard researchers. Retrospective, 2,622 former college athletes, 2,776 controls who were not college athletes. "For all alumnae, a low-milk diet was a risk factor for first bone fracture at or after age 40."

The seven studies showing that milk and dairy consumption during childhood make no difference to fracture risk at any age:

1. Cline, A. D., et al. "Stress Fractures in Female Army Recruits: Implications of Bone Density, Calcium Intake, and Exercise." *Journal of the American College of Nutrition* 17 (1998): 128. Colorado State University researchers. Retrospective, 49 women recruits, ages 18 to 33, who suffered fractures, 78 fracture-free controls. "Fractures in female army recruits were not correlated with bone mineral density or calcium during adolescence."

2. Cumming, R. G., et al. "Case-Control Study of Risk Factors for Hip Fracture in the Elderly." *American Journal of Epidemiology* 139 (1994): 493. Australian researchers. Retrospective, 209 cases, 207 controls. "Consumption of dairy products, particularly at age 20, was associated with an *increased* risk of hip fracture in old age." Compared with participants who consumed the least dairy as children, those who consumed the most suffered *2.9 times as many hip fractures.*

3. Laker, S. R., et al. "Stress Fractures in Elite Cross-Country Athletes." *Orthopedics* 30 (2007): 313. University of Colorado researchers. Retrospective. "Intake of calcium had no statistically significant effect on stress fractures in these athletes."

4. Lofthus, C. M., et al. "Young Patients with Hip Fracture: A Population-Based Study of Bone Mass and Risk Factors for Osteoporosis." *Osteoporosis International* 17 (2006): 1666. Norwegian researchers. Retrospective, 49 cases, ages 20 to 49, compared with Norwegian health data for the same age group. There was no significant difference in calcium intake between the two groups.

5. Loud, K. J., et al. "Correlates of Stress Fracture Among Preadolescent and Adolescent Girls." *Pediatrics* 115 (2005): e399. Harvard researchers. Retrospective, 5,461 girls. "Calcium intake and daily dairy intake were unrelated to stress fractures."

6. Nieves, J. W., et al. "A Case-Control Study of Hip Fracture: Evaluation of Selected Dietary Variables and Teenage Physical Activity." *Osteoporosis International* 2 (1992): 122. Columbia University researchers. Retrospective, 161 cases, 168 controls. "No association was found between recent intake of calcium and hip fracture. Also, teenage calcium and milk drinking were not related to hip fracture."

7. Petridou, E., et al. "The Role of Dairy Products and Non-Alcoholic Beverages in Bone Fractures Among Schoolage Children." *Scandinavian Journal of Social Medicine* 25 (1997): 119. Greek researchers. Retrospective, 100 cases, 100 controls. "Intake of dairy products was not related to the occurrence of fractures."

Appendix C
Scorecard: Does Vitamin D, with or Without Calcium, Reduce Fracture Risk?

The seventeen studies showing it does:

1. Bischoff-Ferrari, H. A., et al. "Fracture Prevention with Vitamin D Supplementation: A Meta-Analysis of Randomized Controlled Trials." *Journal of the American Medical Association* 293 (2005): 2257. Harvard researchers. Meta-analysis of 5 vitamin D trials with or without calcium. Fracture risk reduced 23 percent.

2. Boonen, S., et al. "Need for Additional Calcium to Reduce the Risk of Hip Fracture with Vitamin D Supplementation: Evidence from a Comparative Meta-Analysis of Randomized Controlled Trials." *Journal of Clinical Endocrinology and Metabolism* 92 (2007): 1415. Belgian and Harvard researchers. Six trials. Hip fracture risk reduced 18 percent with vitamin D and calcium. No fewer fractures with just vitamin D.

3. Chapuy, M. C., et al. "Combined Calcium and Vitamin D3 Supplementation in Elderly Women: Confirmation of Reversal of Secondary Hyperparathyroidism and Hip Fracture Risk: The Decalyos II Study." *Osteoporosis*

International 13 (2002): 257. French researchers. Prospective, 583 women in nursing homes, average age 85, followed for 2 years. Fractures reduced 69 percent.

4. Chapuy, M. C., et al. "Vitamin D3 and Calcium to Prevent Hip Fracture in Elderly Women." *New England Journal of Medicine* 327 (1992): 1637. French researchers. Prospective, 3,270 women in nursing homes, average age 84, followed for 1.5 years. Fractures reduced 37 percent.

5. Dawson-Hughes, B., et al. "Effect of Calcium and Vitamin D Supplementation on Bone Density in Men and Women 65 Years of Age or Older." *New England Journal of Medicine* 337 (1997): 670. Tufts University researchers. Prospective, 389 men and women over 65 followed for 3 years. Fractures reduced 60 percent.

6. Feskanich, D., et al. "Calcium, Vitamin D, Milk Consumption and Hip Fractures: A Prospective Study Among Postmenopausal Women." *American Journal of Clinical Nutrition* 77 (2003): 504. Harvard researchers. Prospective, 72,337 postmenopausal women followed for 18 years. Milk and calcium did not reduce fractures. Vitamin D by itself reduced fracture risk 37 percent.

7. Gillespie, W. J., et al. "Vitamin D and Vitamin D Analogues for Preventing Fractures Associated with Involutional and Post-Menopausal Osteoporosis." *Cochrane Database Systematic Reviews* CD000227 (2001). New Zealand researchers. Meta-analysis. Fracture risk reduced 54 percent in the general population, 26 percent among nursing home residents.

8. Izaks, G. J. "Fracture Prevention with Vitamin D Supplementation: Considering the Inconsistent Results." *BMC Muskuloskeletal Disorders* 8 (2007): 26. Meta-analysis of 11 trials. Dutch researcher. Fracture risk reduced 12 percent in the general population, 20 percent in nursing home residents.

9. Jackson, C., et al. "The Effect of Cholcalciferol (vitamin D3) on the Risk of Fall and Fracture: A Meta-Analysis." *QJM* 100 (2007): 185. British researchers. Nine studies. Fractures reduced 4 percent in the general population, 19 percent among postmenopausal women.

10. Larsen, E. R., et al. "Vitamin D and Calcium Supplementation Prevents Osteoporotic Fractures in Elderly Community Dwelling Residents: A Pragmatic Population-Based Three-Year Intervention Study." *Journal of Bone and Mineral Research* 19 (2004): 370. Danish researchers. Prospective,

9,605 men and women, aged 66 or older, followed for 3 years. Fractures reduced 16 percent.

11. Orimo, H., et al. "Reduced Occurrence of Vertebral Crush Fractures in Senile Osteoporosis Treated with 1 Alpha (OH)-vitamin D3." *Bone and Mineral* 3 (1987): 47. Japanese researchers. Prospective, 86 elderly people, 22 cases, 25 controls. "Occurrence of spinal crush fractures was significantly less in the vitamin D group."

12. Orimo, H., et al. "Effects of 2 Alpha-Hydroxyvitamin D3 on Lumbar Bone Mineral Density and Vertebral Fractures in Patients with Postmenopausal Osteoporosis." *Calcified Tissues International* 54 (1994): 370. "The vertebral fracture rate was significantly less in the treated group [i.e., those who took vitamin D] than in the control group."

13. Papadimitropoulos, E., et al. "Meta-analysis of Therapies for Postmenopausal Osteoporosis. VIII: Meta-Analysis of the Efficacy of Vitamin D Treatment in Preventing Osteoporosis in Postmenopausal Women." *Endocrinology Review* 23 (2002): 560. International group of researchers. Twenty-five studies. Fracture risk reduced 23 percent.

14. Riggs, B. L., et al. "Effect of the Fluoride/Calcium Regimen on Vertebral Fracture Occurrence in Postmenopausal Osteoporosis. Comparison with Conventional Therapy." *New England Journal of Medicine* 306 (1982): 446. Prospective, 104 postmenopausal women followed for 3.7 years. With vitamin D and calcium, fractures reduced 50 percent.

15. Tang, B. M. P., et al. "Use of Calcium or Calcium in Combination with Vitamin D Supplementation to Prevent Fractures and Bone Loss in People Aged 50 Years and Older: A Meta-Analysis." *Lancet* 370 (2007): 657. Australian researchers. Meta-analysis of 17 trials. Fracture risk reduced 12 percent.

16. Tilyard, M. W., et al. "Treatment of Postmenopausal Osteoporosis with Calcitriol or Calcium." *New England Journal of Medicine* 326 (1992): 357. "The women who received calcitriol [i.e., vitamin D] had a significant reduction in the rate of new vertebral fractures."

17. Trivedi, D. P., et al. "Effect of Four Monthly Oral Vitamin D3 Supplementations on Fractures and Mortality in Men and Women Living in the Community: Randomized Double-Blind Controlled Trial." *BMJ* [formerly

British Medical Journal] 326 (7387) (2003): 469. British researchers. Prospective, 2,686 elderly followed 5 years. Fractures reduced 33 percent.

The three inconclusive trials:

1. Avenell, A., et al. "Vitamin D and Vitamin D Analogues for Preventing Fractures Associated with Involutional and Postmenopausal Osteoporosis." *Cochrane Database of Systematic Reviews* CD000227 (2005). Scottish researchers. Meta-analysis, 33 studies. "Vitamin D showed no statistically significant effect on hip fracture (seven trials, 18,668 participants), vertebral fractures (four trials, 5,698 participants), or any new fracture (eight trials, 18,903 participants). Vitamin D with calcium marginally reduced hip fractures (seven trials, 10,376 participants), and nonvertebral fractures (seven trials, 10,376 participants), but there was no evidence of effect of vitamin D with calcium on vertebral fractures. The effect appeared to be restricted to those living in institutional care [i.e., nursing homes]."

2. Boonen, S., et al. "Need for Additional Calcium to Reduce the Risk of Hip Fracture With Vitamin D Supplementation: Evidence from a Comparative Meta-Analysis of Randomized Controlled Trials." *Journal of Clinical Endocrinology and Metabolism* 92 (2007): 1415. Belgian researchers. Meta-analysis, four trials. Vitamin D alone had no effect on hip fractures. Vitamin D plus calcium reduced hip fracture risk marginally.

3. Shikari, M., et al. "Effects of 2 Years' Treatment of Osteoporosis with 1 Alpha-Hydroxyvitamin D3 on Bone Mineral Density and Incidence of Fracture: A Placebo-Controlled, Double-Blind Prospective Study." *Endocrinology Journal* 43 (1996): 211. Japanese researchers. Prospective, 113 elderly women with osteoporosis followed for 2 years. In the group receiving vitamin D, fractures were reduced 66 percent. But because of the small number of participants, this result was not statistically significant.

The seventeen studies showing no benefit:

1. Gallagher, J. C., and D. Goldgar. "Treatment of Postmenopausal Osteoporosis with High Doses of Synthetic Calcitriol. A Randomized Controlled Study." *Annals of Internal Medicine* 113 (1990): 649. Creighton University researchers, Omaha, Nebraska. Prospective, 50 elderly women followed for 2 years. "There were no differences between the two groups."

2. Grant, A. M., et al. "Oral Vitamin D3 and Calcium for Secondary Prevention of Low-Trauma Fractures in Elderly People (Randomized Evaluation

of Calcium or Vitamin D, the RECORD study): A Randomized, Placebo-Controlled Trial." *Lancet* 365 (9471) (2005): 1621. British researchers. Prospective, 5,292 men and women, aged 70 or older, followed for up to 5 years. "Findings do not support routine supplementation with calcium and vitamin D3, either alone or in combination, for the prevention of fractures in elderly people."

3. Jackson, R. D., et al. "Calcium Plus Vitamin D and the Risk of Fractures." *New England Journal of Medicine* 354 (2006): 669. Ohio State University researchers. Prospective, 36,282 women, ages 50 to 79 at the start, followed for 7 years. "Among healthy postmenopausal women, calcium with vitamin D did not significantly reduce hip fracture."

4. Jackson, C., et al. "The Effect of Cholecalciferol (Vitamin D3) on the Risk of Fall and Fracture: A Meta-Analysis." *QJM* [formerly *Quarterly Journal of Medicine*] 100 (2007): 185. British researchers. Meta-analysis, 9 trials. Vitamin D had no significant effect on fracture risk.

5. Komulainen, M. H., et al. "HRT and Vitamin D in Prevention of Non-Vertebral Fractures in Postmenopausal Women: A Five-Year Randomized Trial." *Maturitas* 31 (1998): 45. Finnish researchers. Prospective, 464 postmenopausal women followed for 5 years. "In the vitamin D group, the fracture incidence was nonsignificantly decreased in comparison with the placebo group."

6. Law, M., et al. "Vitamin D Supplementation and the Prevention of Fractures and Falls: Results of a Randomized Trial in Elderly People in Residential Accommodation." *Age and Ageing* 35 (2006): 482. British researchers. Prospective, 3,717 nursing home residents, average age 85, followed for up to 14 months.

7. Lips, P., et al. "Vitamin D Supplementation and Fracture Incidence in Elderly People. A Randomized, Placebo-Controlled Clinical Trial." *Annals of Internal Medicine* 124 (1996): 400. Dutch researchers. Prospective, 2,578 men and women over 70 followed for 3.5 years, taking either a placebo or vitamin D. The vitamin D group suffered *more* fractures, but this finding was not statistically significant. "Our results do not show a decrease in the incidence of hip fractures and other peripheral fractures in Dutch elderly persons after vitamin D supplementation."

8. Loud, K. J., et al. "Correlates of Stress Fractures Among Preadolescent and Adolescent Girls." *Pediatrics* 115 (2005): e399. Harvard researchers.

Retrospective, 5,461 girls, ages 11 to 17. "Calcium intake, vitamin D intake, and daily dairy intake were all unrelated to stress fractures."

9. Lyons, R. A., et al. "Preventing Fractures Among Older People Living in Institutional Care: A Pragmatic Randomized Double-Blind Placebo-Controlled Trial of Vitamin D Supplementation." *Osteoporosis International* 18 (2007): 811. British researchers. Prospective, 3,440 elderly men and women followed for 3 years. "Supplementation with oral vitamin D is not sufficient to affect fracture incidence among older people living in institutional care."

10. Meyer, H. E., et al. "Can Vitamin D Supplementation Reduce the Risk of Fracture in the Elderly? A Randomized Controlled Trial." *Journal of Bone and Mineral Research* 17 (2002): 709. Norwegian researchers. Prospective, 1,144 nursing home residents followed for 2 years. "We found that 10 micrograms of vitamin D3 alone produced no fracture-preventive effect in a nursing home population."

11. Michaelsson, K., et al. "Dietary Calcium and Vitamin D Intake in Relation to Osteoporotic Fracture Risk." *Bone* 32 (2003): 694. Swedish researchers. Prospective, 60,689 women, ages 40 to 74 at the start, followed for 11 years. "Dietary calcium or vitamin D intakes estimated at middle age and older age do not seem to be of major importance for the primary prevention of osteoporotic fractures."

12. Munger, R. G., et al. "Prospective Study of Dietary Protein Intake and Risk of Hip Fracture in Postmenopausal Women." *American Journal of Clinical Nutrition* 69 (1999): 147. Utah State University researchers. Prospective, 41,837 postmenopausal Iowa women followed for 3 years. "The risk of hip fracture was not related to intake of calcium or vitamin D."

13. Ott, S. M., and C. H. Chestnut. "Calcitriol Treatment is Not Effective in Postmenopausal Osteoporosis." *Annals of Internal Medicine* 110 (1989): 267. University of Washington, Seattle, researchers. Prospective, 86 postmenopausal women followed for 2 years. "New fractures were seen in 16 percent of the placebo group and 26 percent of the calcitriol [i.e., vitamin D] group." In other words, vitamin D increased fracture risk.

14. Porthouse, J., et al. "Randomized Controlled Trial of Calcium and Supplementation with Cholecalciferol (Vitamin D3) for Prevention of Fracture in Primary Care." *BMJ* [formerly *British Medical Journal*] 330 (7498)

(2005): 1003. British researchers. Prospective, 3,314 women, aged 70 or older, followed for up to 3.5 years. "We found no evidence that calcium and vitamin D supplementation reduces the risk of clinical fractures in women with one or more risk factors for hip fracture."

15. Richy, F., et al. "Efficacy of Alphacalcidol and Calcitriol in Primary and Corticosteroid-Induced Osteoporosis: A Meta-Analysis of Their Effects on Bone Mineral Density and Fracture Rate." *Osteoporosis International* 15 (2004): 301. Belgian researchers. Meta-analysis, 17 studies. "Only two studies specifically addressed the effects of calcitriol on spinal fracture rate. Neither provided significant results."

16. Smith, H., et al. "Effect of Annual Intramuscular Vitamin D on Fracture Risk in Elderly Men and Women: A Population-based, Randomized, Double-Blind, Placebo-Controlled Trial." *Rheumatology* 46 (2007): 1852. British researchers. Prospective, 9,440 men and women over 75 followed for 3 years. "Annual injection of 300,000 IU of vitamin D2 is not effective in preventing non-vertebral fractures among elderly men and women in the general population."

17. Wooton, R., et al. "Fractured Neck of Femur in the Elderly: An Attempt to Identify Patients at Risk." *Clinical Sciences* 57 (1979): 93. Retrospective, 110 cases, 72 controls. "A striking finding was the marked similarity of all variables [blood levels of calcium and vitamin D] in the fracture and control groups."

References

References to the twelve hundred studies that form the basis of this book can be found at www.BuildingBoneVitality.com.

Abstracts of all the studies can be obtained for FREE from the National Library of Medicine's PubMed service's website (www.pubmed.gov):

- On the home page left navigation bar, click Single Citation Matcher.
- Here is a sample citation: Lanou, A. J., et al. "Calcium, Dairy Products, and Bone Health in Children and Young Adults: A Re-Evaluation of the Evidence." *Pediatrics* 115 (2005): 736.

  "Lanou AJ" is the author.
  "Calcium . . . Evidence" is the title.
  "*Pediatrics*" is the journal.
  "115" is the volume.
  "2005" is the year of publication.
  "736" is the first page of the article.

- On the Single Citation Matcher page, fill in the journal, year, volume, first page, author, and one or more key words from the article title. Note: It's rarely necessary to provide all this information. Quite often the journal, year, volume, and first page are enough. Other partial combinations work too.

Or, if you prefer, we're happy to send you copies of all twelve-hundred-plus abstracts plus other documentation, 1,536 pages in all. The documentation package weighs 20 pounds. We ship via UPS to business or residential street addresses. No PO boxes. The cost for copying, shipping, and handling: $250. No credit cards. Check or money order only. Payable to: Self-Care Associates, PO Box 460066, San Francisco, CA 94146. Allow three weeks.

Index

Page numbers followed by "f" or "t" refer to figures or tables respectively.

About the Authors

Amy Joy Lanou, Ph.D., is an assistant professor of health and wellness at the University of North Carolina, Asheville. She has taught nutrition at Cornell University and Ithaca College. She is the author of *Healthy Eating for Life for Children* (Wiley, 2002). She has written or delivered more than fifty scientific articles, reports, and presentations, with an emphasis on bone health and the benefits of low-acid eating. In 2005, she testified before the committee that revised the USDA Food Pyramid and urged the members to embrace the low-acid approach. They didn't. She is also a senior nutrition scientist for the Physicians Committee for Responsible Medicine, a Washington, D.C.–based nonprofit organization dedicated to promoting preventive medicine through nutrition. Dr. Lanou received her B.S. in Nutrition Science from the University of California at Davis (1985) and her Ph.D. in Human Nutrition from Cornell University (1994).

Michael Castleman, M.A., has been called "one of the nation's top health writers" (*Library Journal*). Over the past thirty-five years, he has written more than fifteen hundred health articles for national magazines, plus twelve consumer health books, including *An Aspirin a Day, Nature's Cures, Before You Call the Doctor,* and *The Healing Herbs*, which has sold more than a million copies. He has been nominated for National Magazine Awards twice, for articles on advances in breast cancer prevention, detection, and treatment and how smoking destroys the body. He is a Phi Beta Kappa graduate of the University of Michigan (1972). He earned a master's degree in journalism at UC Berkeley (1979) and has taught medical writing at the Graduate School of Journalism there. He lives in San Francisco. Visit mcastleman.com.